Experimental Skin Grafts and Transplantation Immunity

Donald L. Ballantyne
John Marquis Converse

Experimental Skin Grafts and Transplantation Immunity

A RECAPITULATION

With 60 illustrations

Springer-Verlag
New York   Heidelberg   Berlin

Donald L. Ballantyne, Ph.D.
Professor of Experimental Surgery
New York University School of Medicine
Chief, Microsurgical Research and Training Laboratories
Institute of Reconstructive Plastic Surgery
New York University Medical Center
550 First Avenue
New York, New York 10016/U.S.A.

John Marquis Converse, M.D.
Lawrence D. Bell Professor of Plastic Surgery
New York University School of Medicine
Director, Institute of Reconstructive Plastic Surgery
New York University Medical Center
550 First Avenue
New York, New York 10016/U.S.A.

Library of Congress Cataloging in Publication Data

Ballantyne, Donald L
  Experimental skin grafts and transplantation immunity.

  Bibliography: p.
  Includes index.
  1. Skin-grafting. 2. Transplantation immunology. I. Converse, John
Marquis, joint author. II. Title.
QR188.8.B34   617'.477   79-16175

Softcover reprint of the hardcover 1st edition 1979

9 8 7 6 5 4 3 2 1

ISBN-13: 978-1-4612-6225-1   e-ISBN-13: 978-1-4612-6223-7
DOI: 10.1007/ 978-1-4612-6223-7

Preface

The skin allograft has been used as the test tool since the beginning of investigations of the fate of skin transplanted between two individuals of ordinary genetic diversity. This monograph is designed to furnish the transplantation worker with a review of the significant papers in which skin allografts and xenografts, applied to experimental animals and man, have played a role in acquiring a body of knowledge concerning the behavior and fate of these transplants and the reaction of the body to their presence.

Skin, an essential organ for survival, a barrier between the "milieu interieur" of Claude Bernard and the "milieu exterieur," will remain the most frequently used transplant in transplantation research. Because it is highly antigenic, the final solution of the problem of acceptance of allografts of various tissues and organs will probably depend upon the achievement of a permanent survival of skin allografts.

My personal interest in transplantation, which originated during my surgical training, was rekindled when I met Peter Medawar (today Sir Peter) in England during World War II. I had joined, in 1940, an American Volunteer Surgical Unit (The American Hospital in Britain), organized and headed by Dr. Philip D. Wilson, Surgeon in Chief of the Hospital for Special Surgery in New York. The Unit established an Orthopaedic Center in the Park Prewett Hospital in Basingstoke, Hampshire, adjacent to the Plastic Surgery Center of Sir Harold Gillies. While I was skin grafting the burned face of a pilot of the Battle of Britain, Sir Harold Gillies introduced me to a tall masked young man, Peter Medawar, a zoologist from Oxford University, who watched me operating and began asking questions concerning skin "homografts." He wondered whether the epidermis, separated from the dermis by trypsin, might survive as an allograft. He left, taking with him a piece of the split-thickness skin graft. When the layer of epidermis was subsequently layed upon a granulating wound, alas, it promptly melted away.

Medawar persisted in his research, publishing a series of momentous papers in 1944 and subsequent years (see References); he demonstrated the accelerated rejection of a second-set skin allograft, thus suggesting that allograft rejection was caused by an immunological response to the foreign transplant. New hope arose that "the homograft problem" could be solved. A revival of interest began despite the pessimistic conclusion of the extensive research by Leo Loeb, compiled in his book, *The Biological Basis of Individuality*, in 1945, that an individuality differential limited the possibility of a solution.

After my return from the war in 1946 I resumed by position as a member of the faculty of the Department of Surgery of the New York University School of Medicine. In 1949 Dr. Blair O. Rogers, who coincidentally had an interest in the "homograft problem," stimulated by Dr. Jerome P. Webster at Columbia University, joined the staff as a surgical resident. He wrote an extensive review of the subject in *Plastic and Reconstructive Surgery* in 1951. In 1952 we were able to expand our research activities as the result of a grant from the Atomic Energy Commission, the first grant in the United States for transplantation research. Dr. Donald L. Ballantyne joined our research group in 1954.

A number of early contributions originated from this project; one was that of two or our collaborators, Taylor and Lehrfeld (1953), who discovered that the onset of the rejection phenomenon could be pinpointed by the stereomicroscopic observation of the cessation of hemic flow in the blood vessels of a skin allograft. This test played an important role in defining the rejection time of experimental skin allografts in man, and in subsequent cell transfer experiments in collaboration with Drs. Felix T. Rapaport and H. S. Lawrence and later with Professor Jean Dausset, of the University of Paris, with whom we collaborated in the development of the HLA complex, in man the main histocompatibility complex (MHC).

Dr. Ballantyne has made many contributions to the advancement of knowledge concerning skin transplants; many of these are reviewed in this monograph. The papers reviewed were carefully chosen. Despite careful editing some amount of repetition has been allowed deliberately to avoid numerous referrals to other sections of the text. We hope that by assembling the reviews, workers of various disciplines engaged in transplantation research can obtain the information they seek without having to consult the individual publications.

John Marquis Converse

Acknowledgments

The authors gratefully acknowledge the patience and assistance of Miss Alice D. Harper for her frequent reviewing, checking, and useful suggestions during the course of preparing this book. We are also indebted to Miss Alice Brzytwa, Mrs. Zöe McCullough, and Miss Christine Ahrens for their secretarial work. Many thanks to Ms. Eleonor Pasmik and Ms. Betty Flowers of the New York University Medical Center Library for their bibliographic assistance in connection with the preparation of this monograph.

The senior author would like to express his gratitude to his wife, Mary Lou Ballantyne, for her deep interest, encouragement, and aid in the preparation of this book.

Contents

Introduction

This review is concerned with a wide variety of theories on the nature of reparative changes, including the mode of vascularization, and the subsequent biologic events that determine the behavior and eventual fate of skin grafts. Special attention has been given to the clinical and experimental lines of evidence supporting the theories of the vascularization process of different types of grafts. In addition, the development of various diagnostic methods to establish criteria for the evaluation of graft survival end points and the theories underlying the mechanisms responsible for the demise of allografts are reviewed and discussed.

Although it is general knowledge that almost without exception the exchanges of skin between genetically unrelated individuals of the same species do not survive long, a search of the literature shows no comprehensive review of the sequential events from the time of complete revascularization to the survival end point of the grafts. Furthermore, there is no review pertaining to skin grafts removed from one species and transplanted to another, despite reports indicating a very restricted survival time in these grafts.

No attempt will be undertaken to review the entire body of literature concerning the immunogenetic complexities of transplantation immunity and its mechanism of action on the grafts. However, it seems necessary to provide an introductory outline of the nomenclature that describes each type of skin graft, its pertinent properties, and conditions of survival. Also included is a brief description of the characteristics of transplantation that account for unexpected deviations from the normal course of skin graft behavior and survival times. This information is important for a better understanding of the possible interactions between the vascular system of the skin graft, the cytologic alterations occurring within the cellular and fibrous structures of the skin graft, and the timing and intensity of the immune response.

Types of Grafts and Their General Properties

Current descriptive terms are used to define types of grafts (Gorer 1960; Gorer, Loutit, and Micklem 1961; Medawar 1962; Snell 1964; Russell and Monaco 1965): *autograft* designates a graft in which the donor is also the recipient; *allograft* (formerly homograft) describes a graft exchanged between genetically unrelated members of the same species or between different inbred strains; and *xenograft* (formerly heterograft) indicates that the transplantation of tissue or organ was between individuals of different species, e.g., man to dog, or rat to rabbit. The term *isograft* is usually used to denote an allograft between normal members of genetically highly uniform strains of the same animal species. These animals are referred to as *inbred* or *isogenic* strains.

When a tissue graft is applied to a recipient for the first time, it is defined as either a *primary* or *first-set graft*. *Second-set grafts* are grafts transplanted to the same recipients that have already received prior grafts from the same donor.

Skin autografts are always successful and survive permanently in the new environment, known as the *recipient* or *host* bed, if careful preoperative, surgical, and postoperative procedures are applied and the restoration of an adequate blood supply is assured. On the other hand, allografts are usually rejected after the host has made a semblance of accepting them during the first 5 or 6 days. During this limited period of survival, allografts resemble autografts, exhibiting similar cellular proliferation and activity, but they are eventually destroyed when the immune mechanisms elicited by the presence of foreign tissue become fully developed. The typical breakdown of a normal tissue or tumor from a genetically dissimilar individual of the same species is referred to as an *allograft rejection*.

Tissue isografts interchanged between members of the same isogenic strain of mice react like autografts and may survive permanently. Isografts evoke fewer and milder immune responses in their recipients than do allografts of similar tissue. An important exception to the rule of permanent survival of skin grafts exchanged between members of a strictly inbred mouse strain was discovered by Eichwald and Silmser in 1955. In most isogenic mouse strains, skin grafts from males to females are rejected, whereas the isografts between similar sexes or from females to males succeed permanently. The immune response evoked by male grafts in female recipients has been attributed by Eichwald, Silmser, and Wheeler (1957) to the histocompatibility gene associated with the nonpairing segment of the Y chromosome.

In humans the donor and host must be identical (monozygotic) twins for skin transplants to behave like autografts and survive a long time or permanently (Padgett 1932; Brown 1937; Converse and Duchet 1947; Blandford and Garcia 1953; Rogers 1957a, b, 1959; Rogers and Bach 1964). Allogeneic skin, when exchanged between dizygotic cattle twins, reacts in an auto-graftlike fashion and survives for long periods of time, sometimes even permanently, whereas grafts between bovine siblings of independent birth are rejected in the normal fashion (Owen 1945; Anderson, Billingham, Lampkin, and Medawar 1951; Billingham, Lampkin, Medawar, and Williams 1952). This type of induced tolerance of skin grafts in cattle has been attributed by the authors to erythrocyte chimerism,[1] a result of vascular anastomoses between the embryos in utero.

Xenografts have a restricted survival time and are destroyed more rapidly and violently than allografts (Woodruff 1960; Russell and Monaco 1965; Ben-Hur, Solowey, and Rapaport 1969a, b; Ben-Hur 1974). The severity of the host's immunologic defense mechanisms evoked by xenogeneic tissue is more readily evident when compared with the response to allografts. The very rapidity (minutes to hours) of some xenograft reactions probably reflects the presence of heterophile antibodies[2] and antigens with some elements of host presensitization.

With the development by Padgett (1939) of the dermatome and other mechanical cutting devices for removing skin grafts, it is possible to obtain grafts of varying thickness. The thin skin graft was named after the German surgeon Thiersch in 1874, and is also referred to as the Ollier-Thiersch graft, after the French surgeon who also described a technique for the removal of larger grafts. It includes only the epidermis and a thin layer of the dermis, while the split-thickness graft consists of one-third to three-quarters the thickness of the subjacent dermal layer (Padgett 1939). The full-thickness graft, also known as the Wolfe (1875) graft, extends to the subcutaneous layer.

Most investigators, working with laboratory animals, have used different types of grafts. In one type, the *suprapannicular* graft, the skin graft is removed from above the panniculus carnosus, the thin discontinuous muscular membrane separating the dermis from the deeper underlying tissues. In the other, the *subpannicular* graft, the skin, together with the panniculus, is removed. The panniculus carnosus is well developed in most animals; in man it is represented by the platysma muscle layer beneath the cervical skin.

Immunologic Mechanisms of the Rejection Response

In defining the local events connected with allograft rejection, Loeb (1945) has been credited with the concept that there are basic differences in the chemical structure between the graft and the host, which he termed *indi-*

---

[1] Chimera: an individual composed of genetically dissimilar tissue.

[2] Heterophile antibodies: antibodies that react against heterophile antigens, which are antigens shared by more than one species.

viduality differentials. Medawar (1944) showed that the allograft reaction was an immunologic reaction by demonstrating the second-set phenomenon. This is an accelerated rejection which occurs when a second allograft, of either a similar or dissimilar tissue, from the same donor is applied to the same recipient after the destruction of a first graft. Medawar (1958) attributed to Jensen (1903) the inception of the idea that the allogeneic rejection is mediated by a process of *active immunity*. Jensen used the term "active immunity" to describe the process by which a transplanted tumor in the mouse is first accepted and then rejected by the host. The allograft rejection reaction is a readily observable response which shows many of the gross aspects of an immunologic process. An impressive array of experimental data supports this immunologic hypothesis (Russell and Winn 1970).

With the advent of inbred and congenic resistant strains of mice, it soon became obvious that the delicate balance between rejection and survival of grafted tissue depends on autosomal dominant genes that control the immunologic response to specific antigens. Indeed, extensive systematic genetic studies with mice by many authorities, including Gorer (1942), Snell (1948, 1953, 1958), Barnes and Krohn (1957), and McKhann (1964), indicate that the severity and the speed of the host's reaction against tumors and grafted normal tissues, including skin, are influenced by the immunogenetic differences between donor and host. The antigenic differences involved in transplantation immunity are determined by dominant genes (Gorer 1938), which were termed *histocompatibility genes* by Snell (1948), and which many authors have considered as either "strong" or "weak." Indeed, the histocompatibility genes responsible for the antigenic differences determine the behavior, survival, and eventual breakdown of the tissue grafts; the host responds to the dominant genes present in the donor's tissue but absent in the host's own tissue. Many investigative studies, using inbred and congenic resistant strains of mice, have shown that grafts between strains differing at strong histocompatibility gene loci, known as H-2, are rapidly and violently destroyed (Counce, Smith, Barth, and Snell 1956), whereas differences between the weak histocompatibility loci, such as H-1, H-3, and H-4, may allow longer graft survival (Counce *et al.* 1956; Barnes and Krohn 1957; Winn, Stevens, and Snell 1958; Snell and Stevens 1961). As Berrian and McKhann wrote in 1960, "the variations may reflect differences in the quality and quantity of antigens elaborated by the genes, in their distribution and attachments of immunity in the compatible host." Snell (1971) defined histocompatibility genes as those genes whose end products are cell surface antigens that determine the acceptance or rejection of transplants.

It should also be noted that similar studies involving evidence of histocompatibility in the presence of genetic differences between the donor and recipient have been undertaken in man by Rogers (1963), Rogers and Bach (1964), and Bach and Amos (1967), among others, and likewise in subhuman primates by Gabb, Piazza, d'Amaro, and Balner (1972) and many others.

Much of the information on the immunogenetics of transplantation has also been derived from species other than mice, such as rats (Billingham and Silvers 1959; Billingham, Hodge, and Silvers 1962; White and Hildemann 1968), minipigs (Sachs, Leight, Cone, Schwartz, Stuart, and Rosenberg 1976; Leight, Sachs, and Rosenberg 1977; Leight, Kirkman, Rasmusen, Rosenberg, Sachs, Terrill, and Melville 1978), rabbits (Medawar 1944; Tissot and Cohen 1972; Chai 1974), fish (Hildemann and Haas 1960), amphibians (Cohen 1971), and even birds (Billingham, Brent, and Medawar 1953).

For readers who are interested in more comprehensive and detailed information on the pathogenetic and immunologic mechanisms involved in transplantation biology, excellent reviews by Snell (1957), Brent (1958), Medawar (1958), H. S. Lawrence (1959), Stetson (1963), Russell and Winn (1970) and Billingham and Silvers (1971) are recommended.

Factors That May Influence the Normal Course of Graft Behavior and Survival Time

Mention should be made of the fact that there are certain situations in which skin or solid tissue allografts between genetically dissimilar individuals of the same species can circumvent the histocompatibility barrier and enjoy longer periods of survival. In some instances they may survive permanently. Such variations in immunologic response to grafts have been observed by several authors, among them Billingham and Hildemann (1958a, b), Hildemann and Walford (1960), and Rogers, Raisbeck, Ballantyne, and Converse (1960). There is general agreement that in normal hosts and without any chemotherapeutic or immunosuppressive measures, the variations in immunologic response to allogeneic grafts, as explained by Billingham (1959), depend on a variety of conditions, some of which will be illustrated briefly in the succeeding sections.

Site of Sensitization

Skin allografts placed in privileged recipient sites, such as the cheek pouch of the hamster (Billingham and Silvers 1962) or the anterior chamber of the eye of the rabbit (Medawar 1948; Billingham and Boswell 1953; Greene 1955; Raju and Grogan 1969a), may enjoy long periods of survival in an autograftlike condition. Similar observations with skin grafts in the anterior chamber of the eye of inbred rats across both major and minor histocompatibility barriers were subsequently made by Kaplan and Stevens in 1975. Their results are at variance with those of Franklin and Prendergast (1970), who expressed doubt that the anterior chamber of the rabbit's eye extends an immunologically privileged status to skin grafts, but Kaplan and Stevens attribute the variation in results to animal species, variation in graft size, and other nonspecific factors.

In a subsequent study, Subba Rao and Grogan (1977), working with the anterior chamber of the rat eye, have confirmed and extended the observations of Kaplan and Stevens that the persistence of an auricular skin allograft placed in the anterior chamber is directly associated with the graft size. The findings show that smaller grafts (approximately 0.5 mm² in size) survive significantly longer than larger grafts (approximately 2.0 mm² in size). Subba Rao and Grogan also reported that the pattern and extent of the host response to subsequent orthotopic skin allografts depend on the size of the primary skin grafts within the anterior chamber of the eye. According to them, smaller primary skin allografts are capable of reducing, inhibiting, or delaying the immune response of the animal recipient to further skin challenges from the same donor, thus enhancing the graft survival. In contrast, larger allografts elicit heightened specific resistance in the recipient against further applications of a skin allograft from the same donor, whereby the test grafts are destroyed in an accelerated fashion (see Chapter 7).

Prior to the report of Warden, Reemtsma, and Steinmuller (1973), it was generally accepted that the nature of the privileged site is associated with the fact that neither the cheek pouch of the hamster nor the anterior chamber of the animal eye have any direct lymphatic drainage pathways. However, from the studies of Raju and Grogan (1969a), Warden *et al.* (1973), Kaplan and Stevens (1975), Subba Rao and Grogan (1977), and others, it appears that the persistent survival of allografts in privileged sites is not only due to lack of lymphatic drainage pathways but also to several other possible factors. These possibilities include adaptation of the host to grafts, development of enhancing antibodies, interference with or immunosuppression of cell-mediated antibody, alteration of central processing of the antigen, and inhibition of humoral antibody in the host. When a graft is transplanted to a privileged recipient site, the grafting procedure is said to be *heterotopic,* which means that a graft is transferred to an anatomically different host bed; for example, grafts of skin, cartilage, or adipose tissue to the brain or the eye chamber. An *orthotopic* graft is one placed in an identical topographic host site, such as skin to skin or cartilage to cartilage.

Experimental lines of evidence in support of this interpretation of the role of lymphatic pathways were provided by Barker and Billingham (1967, 1968), who showed that intact lymphatic drainage is necessary for the sensitization of the host to orthotopic skin allografts. By placing grafts on an alymphatic flap of skin whose vascular connection with its host was preserved for blood supply and metabolic exchanges, these authors were able to sustain graft survival in the guinea pig as long as the regrowth of lymphatics could be impeded. This was achieved by dissecting a single artery and vein to an isolated skin flap, which was then placed in a plastic cup fitted with an opening for the vascular pedicle. This island flap of skin then served as a bed for skin grafts, which persisted for as long as the reestablishment of lymphatic connections between the graft and the host was prevented by the physical barrier of the plastic cup.

In conclusion, the experiments by Hall (1967) in sheep and by Barker and Billingham in guinea pigs suggest that, as far as the initial sensitization of the host to orthotopic foreign skin is concerned, an intact lymphatic drainage system together with intact regional lymph nodes is essential. On the other hand, according to Hall (1967), Barker and Billingham (1968), and Billingham and Barker (1969), in the case of organ allografts (or even xenografts) whose blood supply is immediately restored by surgical vascular anastomosis, intact lymphatic drainage is not mandatory for the development of sensitivity.

Animal Species

In 1956, Adams, Patt, and Lutz found that, unlike orthotopic skin allografts studied in most animal species and man, skin allografts exchanged between noninbred members of the same hamster colonies can survive for long periods of time even when the donor and host are not related. Furthermore, Billingham and Hildemann (1958a, b), confirming the findings of Adams and associates, found that in certain colony strain combinations the skin cross-grafted between hamsters obtained from different sources had a prolonged survival, often surviving over 1 year. Similar results have been observed by Hildemann (1957) in goldfish.

Prolongation of Graft Survival Under a Variety of Circumstances

Most skin allografts between unrelated individuals of the same species persist as intact soft tissue for 6–12 days before being rapidly and violently destroyed by the immunologic response of the host, termed the *acute rejection reaction*. Under certain conditions, however, the rejection process can be delayed or modified, permitting graft survival. Sparrow (1953), credited with the first systematic study of skin graft behavior in the guinea pig, found an unexpectedly wide variation in allograft survival time, ranging from 5 to 17 days; one graft persisted to the 45th day, despite the difference in coat color and genetic relationship between the donor and host. There are several other reports in the literature in which normal tissue allografts sometimes showed unexpected prolonged survival although the donor and host were relatively unrelated and unmodified by a specific immunosuppressive or therapeutic treatment.

Variations of a slower, *chronic rejection phenomenon* have been described by many clinicians and experimental workers, including Billingham and Medawar (1951) in various species, Pfeffer and Rogers (1955) in human subjects, and Barnes and Krohn (1957) in mice. In addition, mention should be made of the fact that, apart from the degree of antigenic differences between the individuals and induced graft tolerance by immunologic and drug treatment, changes in graft survival times can be effected by means of irradiation, environmental temperature, and other physical procedures. By cooling a small rat skin graft in situ to approximately 16°C for the first 24 hours after grafting by means of a portable in vivo cooling unit, Daniller, Ballantyne, and Converse (1971) produced a chronic rejection pattern even though transplantation was performed across a strong histocompatibility barrier. The graft survival was changed from a combined average survival of 10 days to a combined average survival of 20 days. Similarly, survival of allogeneic skin across a strong histocompatibility barrier has been reported to be significantly prolonged by physical trauma produced by a severe thermal injury in rabbits (Bailey, Lewis, and Blocker 1962), rats (Rapaport, Converse, Horn, Ballantyne, and Mulholland 1964), mice (Markley, Thornton, and Smallman 1971), and humans (Munster, Eurenius, Katz, Canales, Foley, and Mortensen 1973; Ninnemann, Fisher, and Frank 1978), by a tourniquet injury in mice (Markley *et al.* 1971), and by the application of surgical clips in rats (Markley and Thornton 1973). Prolonged survival of skin allografts in patients with advanced cancer was also reported (Snyderman, Miller, and Lizardo 1960; Gardner and Preston 1962; Graham and Petersons 1965). This effect has been attributed, as in burns, to a breakdown of the recipient's immune response.

A set of useful terms has been provided by Hildemann and Walford (1960) and Rogers (1963) to define variations in the rejection process and in the survival time range of grafted tissue. If an allograft is not rejected acutely or violently, it may undergo one or two possible reactions: (1) a chronic reaction with delayed onset and a prolonged period of rejection; or (2) a long-term persistence of survival in which the graft shrinks gradually from its margins until it attains its survival end point as a fine *linear scar*. In the Syrian hamster, Hildemann and Walford (1960) have subdivided the chronic rejection reaction into three arbitrary categories: *rapid chronic, intermediate chronic,* and *prolonged chronic rejection*. Their observations on the reactivity times of first-set allografts demonstrating a chronic rejection reaction, revealed this general relationship: "the later the time of the onset, the longer the interval between the onset and the survival endpoint."

Quantity of Skin

Considerable attention has been given to the variations in recipient immune response generated by varying the size of skin allografts. According to Medawar (1944), in rabbits the period of survival of grafts varies inversely with their size. With the open-style grafts, which are distributed over the host bed in such a way as to be separated adequately from each other and also from the margins of the adjacent host skin, comparisons between high-dosage grafts with a cumulative weight of 0.36–0.44 g and low-dosage grafts weighing 0.006 g showed median survival times of 10.4 and 15.1 days, respectively. Lehrfeld and Taylor (1953) reported a definite and significant difference in the duration of skin allografts of various sizes in the rat. Large transplants, ranging in size between 100 and 625 mm^2, are rejected in 8 days, whereas the small pinch grafts 1–2 mm in diameter persisted for 21 days before succumbing to immunologic attack. Zotikov, Budik, and Puza (1960), on the other hand, demonstrated that in rats massive skin allografts representing one-third of the body surface of the animal host survive longer than smaller controls.

Further evidence substantiating the data of Zotikov and his associates has been found in many more recent studies, including those of Ballantyne, Siegel, and Kapitchnikov (1962), Converse, Siegel, and Ballantyne (1962, 1963), and Calnan and Kukatilake (1962). The nature of the immune mechanisms underlying the delayed rejection or temporary tolerance of such grafts remains unknown, although the temporary massive destruction of draining lymphatics to regional lymph nodes can be postulated as playing a role. On the other hand, Veith, Murray, and Miller (1966) were unable to obtain prolonged survival of massive full-thickness allografts in dogs, even under immunosuppressive therapy.

Chapter 1

Vascularization of Skin Grafts: Autografts and Allografts

The biologic fate of skin grafts has intrigued clinicians and researchers since the early experiments of Bert (1865). The summary of clinical research observations presented in this chapter is derived mainly from a review by Converse, McCarthy, Brauer, and Ballantyne (1977), incorporating pertinent information from Clemmesen (1967) and Šmahel (1977).

Transplantation of living tissues involves the surgical removal of viable cells from a donor area and subsequent transfer to a recipient site. Whether or not the transplanted cells survive and propagate a lineage of living cells in the recipient site depends on the following factors: (1) the accessibility of nutritive materials; (2) the resources for disposing of metabolic waste products; (3) the anatomic distinction between the tissue of the donor and recipient; and (4) the taxonomic and immunogenetic relationships between the donor and recipient.

Skin, because it is so accessible, has enjoyed considerable attention as a transplantation model and has been extensively investigated. Much of our basic understanding of the biologic laws of tissue transplantation and vascular changes has been derived primarily from the study of skin grafts.

At the time of surgical excision from its donor area, a graft of skin is completely severed from the surrounding skin and subcutaneous tissue layer; the circulation, lymphatic drainage, and nerve continuity are abruptly terminated. It is recognized that the survival of a skin graft is dependent on rapidly acquiring a blood supply adequate for nutrition and for disposal of metabolic waste products. In the time interval between transplantation and the process of revascularization, survival of the anoxic graft cells appears to be maintained by the absorption of fluid from the host (Converse, Ballantyne, Rogers, and Raisbeck 1957; Converse, Uhlschmid, and Ballantyne 1969). This process of imbibition of exudate from the host bed, first noted by Hübscher in 1888 and Goldmann in 1890 and termed by them "plasmatische Zirculation" (plasmatic circulation), appears to play an important role in ensuring an interim period of nourishment before the establishment of a definitive vasculature; however, it is not capable of indefinitely maintaining the survival of a graft, which will eventually perish if it does not become successfully vascularized.

The mode of vascularization of skin grafts is still a subject of debate. Revascularization of skin grafts has been attributed to one or a combination of three processes: (1) direct connection of the graft and host vessels, referred to as "inosculation" (from the Latin verb *inosculare*, to kiss); (2) ingrowth of host vessels into the endothelial channels of the graft; and (3) penetration of the host vessels into the graft dermis, creating new endothelial channels. The available data supporting the roles of these three processes in the revascularization of various types of skin transplants will be reviewed.

The following conditions are necessary for the success of a skin graft: (1) a favorable and well-vascularized host bed; (2) rapid serum imbibition occurring soon after grafting; (3) adequate immobilization of the skin graft on the host site to ensure the exchange of nutrient fluids and to reduce to a minimum any tendency to disrupt delicate newly formed vascular communications between the donor and host; and (4) rapid vascularization from the recipient site.

Phase of Serum Imbibition

Hübscher (1888) and Goldmann (1890) suggested that Thiersch grafts in human patients were nourished by fluid from the host prior to the establishment of new vascular and lymphatic channels in the graft. Using a modification of the tissue chamber technique described by Algire (1943a,b) and Algire and Legallais (1949) for evaluating skin autografts in mice, Conway, Stark, and Joslin (1951) observed a profuse flow of extracellular fluids from the surrounding area of the host into the transparent chamber during the first 24 hours. They stressed the importance of early plasmatic circulation, by which the grafts were able to be sustained during the first postoperative week.

Observations by Converse, Ballantyne, Rogers, and Raisbeck (1957) on a series of skin xenografts removed from the rabbit and placed upon the chorioallantois of the chick embryo indicated a rapid fluid uptake in the graft. The rabbit skin grafts were removed from the surface of the chorioallantoic membrane at time intervals varying from 1 to 20 hours after transplantation. These grafts were weighed prior to transplantation and again after their removal by traction from the membrane. A progressive weight increase with time was observed in 165 grafts (Fig. 1): the average increase in graft weight was 10% after 1 hour, and progressed steadily to 38.2% after 10 hours and to 52% after 20 hours. It has been suggested that a skin graft is capable of absorbing fluid from the host bed because of the spongelike

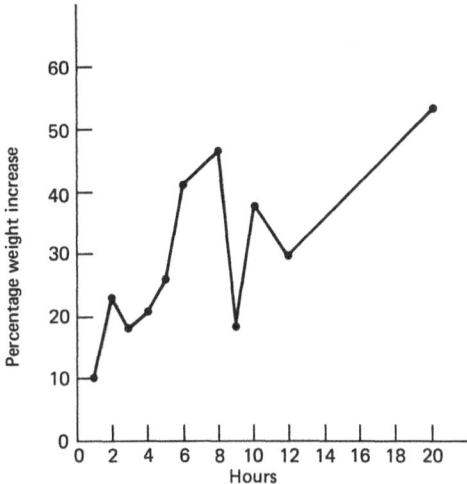

Fig. 1. Weight increase of rabbit skin xenografts 1–20 hours after application to the chorioallantois of chick embryo. Converse, Ballantyne, Rogers, and Raisbeck (1957) Transplant. Bull. 4:154, © (1957) The Williams & Wilkins Co., Baltimore.

structure of the dermis, which is canalized by innumerable endothelial spaces.

Most investigators have generally accepted Hübscher's original concept of plasmatic circulation as an important factor in the early nourishment of skin grafts before the restoration of an adequate blood supply. However, Clemmesen (1962, 1967) believed that the main role of plasmatic circulation is not nutritional. He felt it serves to prevent dessication of the graft and to keep the graft vessels open. Henry, Marshall, Friedman, Dammin, and Merrill (1962), working with human skin grafts, reported that the donor skin derives its nutrition and oxygenation from the process of plasmatic circulation for the first 2 days after grafting. Thereafter, this type of nourishment is inadequate for maintaining the viability of full-thickness grafts, unless it is supplemented by an adequate vascular supply.

Šmahel (1971a, 1977) advanced a theory that the existence, condition, and duration of the phase of plasmatic circulation depend on the following factors: (1) the graft thickness; (2) the length of time a recipient bed is allowed to remain open and heal before the graft is applied; and (3) the lag time between the excision of a skin graft from the donor site and subsequent application to the recipient site.

Biochemical Studies

In a series of experimental studies involving biochemical determinations of skin autografts in the rat, Marckmann and Zachariae (1964) and Marckmann (1965a, b, 1967) studied the response of the graft dermis to injury resulting from the transplantation procedure. During the first 5 critical days, the reaction of a graft to surgical trauma was reflected by edema and changes in the metabolic activity of sulfomucopolysaccharides and in the levels of hexoamine, hydroxyproline, uronic acid, and histamine. These authors assumed that the biochemical alterations in the graft are associated in part with the reduced blood supply, accompanied by changes in the metabolic equilibrium.

Psillakis, de Jorge, Villardo, Albano, Martins, and Spina (1969), after transplanting auricular autografts in rabbits, measured water and electrolyte composition in the graft during the first 5 days. The findings indicated a significant increase in water content (Fig. 2a) on the first day, lasting until the fifth day, whereas the sodium concentration (Fig. 2b), already significantly increased on the first day, showed a subsequent progressive diminution. In contrast, the potassium content (Fig. 2c) was significantly reduced the first 2 days after grafting and increased considerably over the subsequent 3 days. The authors attributed the edema in the graft to the changes in the water and electrolyte levels, which were reflected by the response of collagen to grafting injury, a finding similar to that noted in traumatized tissue. As a consequence of injury, the graft dermis is rich in extracellular macromolecules capable of absorbing water and cations from the recipient site without direct vascular continuity with the host blood supply.

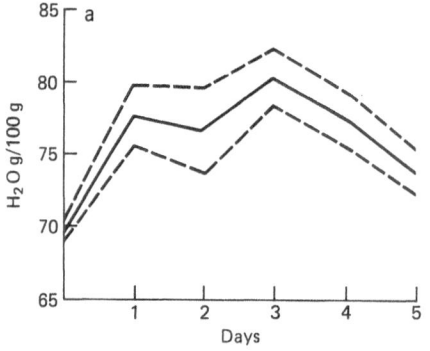 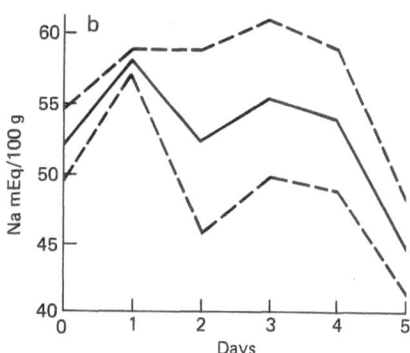

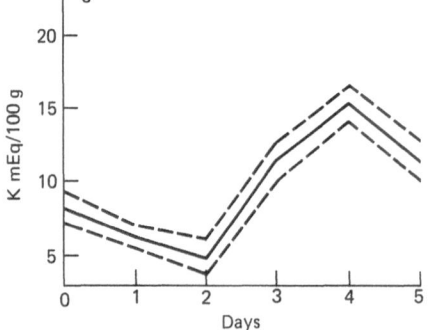

Fig. 2 a–c. Changes in composition of full-thickness skin autografts in rabbits from the first to the fifth day after transplantation. **a.** Water content. **b.** Sodium content. **c.** Potassium content. Psillakis, de Jorge, Villardo, Albano, Martins, and Spina (1969) Plast. Reconstr. Surg. 43:500, © (1969) The Williams & Wilkins Co., Baltimore.

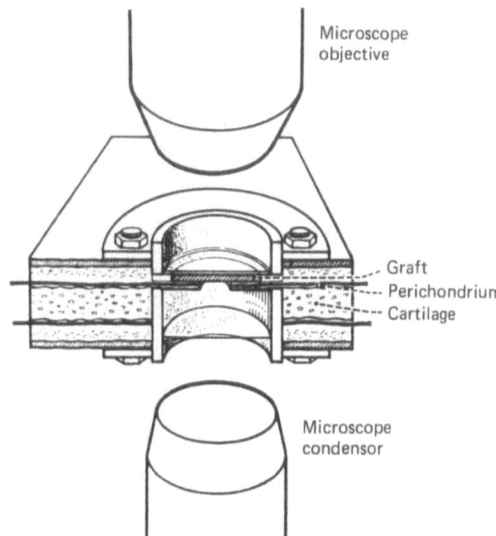

Microscope
objective

Graft
Perichondrium
Cartilage

Microscope
condensor

Fig. 3. Arrangement of free
skin graft inside the rabbit's ear
chamber for vital microscopy.
Birch and Brånemark (1969)
Scand. J. Plast. Surg. 3:1.

Vital Microscopic and Microangiographic Studies

Birch and Brånemark (1969) studied full-thickness scrotal skin autografts
placed on the perichondrial recipient bed of an auricle in rabbits through a
transparent ear chamber by vital microscopy (Fig. 3). They observed graft
edema immediately after grafting. The edema attained its maximum on the
third day after grafting. The authors attributed the edema to the ground
substance depolymerization in the graft dermis, the absorption of tissue
fluids into the graft extracellular compartments, the increased capillary
pressure, and the increased permeability in the inflamed host bed. The
gradual subsidence of the graft edema is due to improved hemodynamics,
which result from the reestablishment of blood and lymphatic circulation. In
a rabbit study using the same transplantation model as well as microangiography, Birch, Brånemark, and Lundskog (1969) reached similar conclusions
concerning the graft edema.

Studies in Experimental Orthotopic Grafts

A study of plasmatic circulation under experimental conditions more closely
approximating the events occurring in orthotopic grafting was undertaken by
Converse, Uhlschmid, and Ballantyne (1969) in the rat. They found a 37.34%
weight gain in full-thickness autografts at 24 hours after grafting, followed
by a decrease in the relative weight gain to 25.69% by 48 hours (Fig. 4). After
this drop, the average weight gain gradually increased again to 30.44% by 96
hours and then steadily returned to its original weight by 9 days. The authors
suggested that the rise in weight between 48 and 72 hours coincided with the

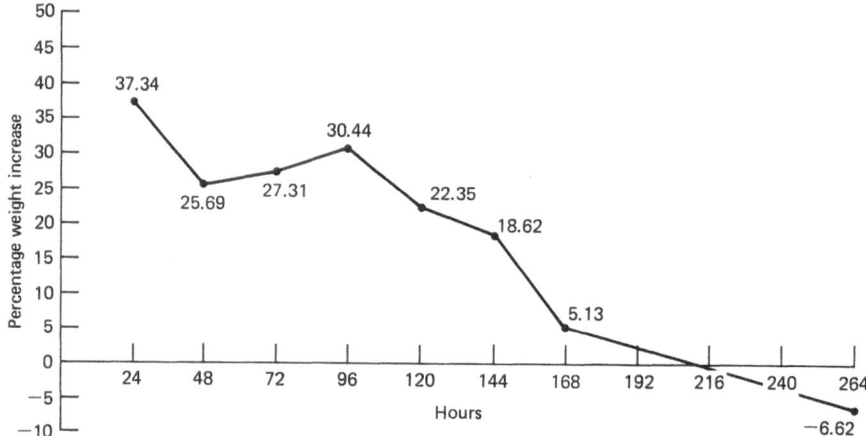

Fig. 4. Percentage of weight increase of rat skin autografts from 24 to 264 hours after transplantation. Converse, Uhlschmid, and Ballantyne (1969) Plast. Reconstr. Surg. 43:495, © (1969) The Williams & Wilkins Co., Baltimore.

development of stereomicroscopically visible blood circulation in the grafts. This weight gain was attributed to the filling of the graft vascular system and the inadequate venous and lymphatic drainage, probably the result of engorgement and interstitial edema. With improved venous drainage subsequent to the establishment of an arterial and venous network, the graft returned to its original weight by 8–9 days following transplantation. The negative values noted on the 11th day may well be attributed to improved venous and lymphatic drainage. The graft is first fixed to the host site by fibrin; thus the fluid penetrating the graft is serum, not plasma. Consequently, it was proposed that the term "plasmatic circulation" be replaced by the term "phase of serum imbibition."

Similar increases in the weight of orthotopic skin grafts, calculated as a percentage of the original graft weight, were obtained by Kubaček (1962), Clemmensen (1967), and Šmahel and Bartos (1967). The relative weight gain of up to 40% during the first few days after transplantation was attributed to the absorption of fluid from the recipient site by the grafts, and the subsequent decrease in the relative weight gain was attributed to the reestablishment of blood circulation in the graft.

Intravenous Colloidal Carbon Suspension Studies

Kikuchi and Omori (1970) injected an intravenous colloidal carbon suspension into rabbits at varying time intervals after full-thickness skin autografting. They reported that during the first 2 days after grafting the principal plasma leakage originated from the venules of the graft bed, although capillaries, terminal arterioles, and metarterioles were also leaking. The phenomenon at the graft–host junction was correlated with the phase of the so-called plasmatic circulation. However, on the third day a different pattern of carbon labeling appeared. It was very faint or even absent, and possibly reflected the change to graft revascularization.

Experiments with the Cheek Pouch of the Syrian Hamster

In order to investigate further the early nutritional process that ensures the viability of a skin graft before the establishment of a definitive vasculature, Haller and Billingham (1964, 1967) and Haller, Rauenhorst, Adkins, and Billingham (1966) selected the cheek pouch of Syrian hamsters (see Fig. 18a and b) as the source of transparent skin grafts. Based on the observations of pouch skin transplanted to the animal flank, the authors attributed the early graft survival to the passive uptake of fluid and erythrocytes from the host bed into the preexisting vessels in the graft. They also termed this process the "phase of imbibition."

Studies on Color Changes in Skin Grafts

When excised from the donor, the graft becomes chalk white and blanched. Within a few hours after transplantation it takes on a pinkish hue and progresses to a bright pink during the next few days. Douglas (1944) noted a faint pink tint in the graft as early as 8 hours after grafting. McLaughlin (1954), studying the color changes in a composite graft of cartilage and skin that had been transferred from the ear to reconstruct the border of a nostril, described a change from blanched white to a more harmonious cutaneous coloration within 6 hours after grafting. Hynes (1954) observed that the blood vessels in freshly cut human skin grafts varying from split thickness to full thickness are collapsed and empty (Fig. 5a). The graft vessels, probably as a result of separation from the donor site, undergo spasm, expelling most of the formed hemic elements through the severed ends of the vessels on the graft undersurface (Fig. 5b). Within 24 hours after transplantation, the graft vessels are again dilated, although they contain only a few hemic elements (Fig. 5c). By 48 hours, the vessels are more distended and contain a large number of erythrocytes (Fig. 5d and e). According to Hynes, the exudate that accumulates at the line of demarcation between the graft and host tissues consists of plasma, numerous erythrocytes, and some polymorphonuclear leukocytes (Fig. 5b). This fluid exudate, after precipitating its fibrinogen in the form of fibrin on the surface of the host site, penetrates the overlying graft vessels as a fibrinogen-free suspension of erythrocytes, thereby nourishing the grafts; this phenomenon is responsible for the rapid color change that occurs within hours of transplantation.

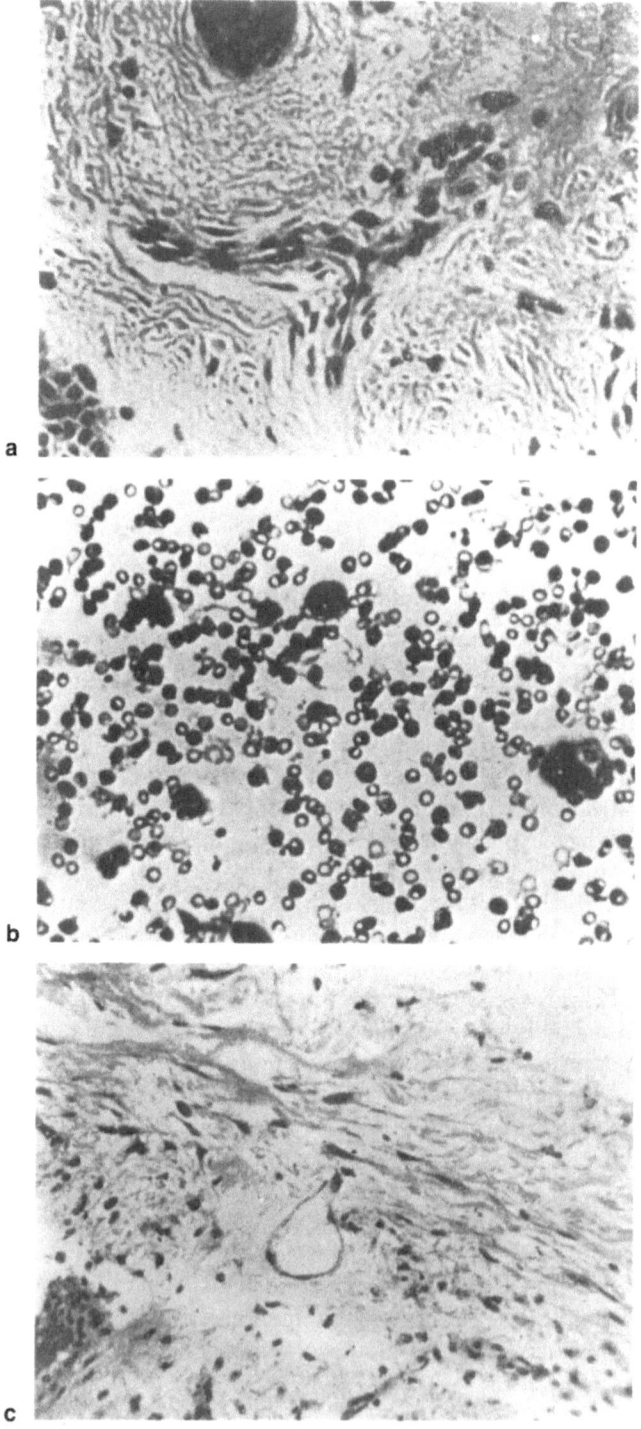

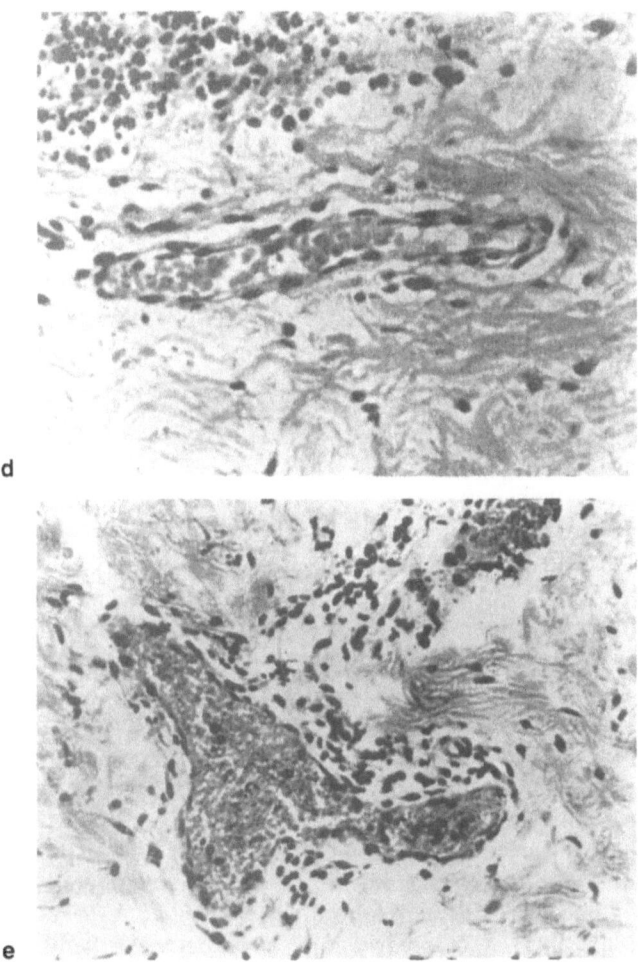

Fig. 5 a–e. Changes in the vessels of a skin graft before, and at various intervals after, it is placed on a healthy granulating defect. **a.** Collapsed empty capillary in the freshly cut skin graft. ×370. **b.** Many red blood cells and some polymorphonuclear leukocytes in the fluid exudate under a skin graft that has been applied to the defect for 24 hours. Leishman's stain. ×240. **c.** Skin graft capillary that is dilated but contains no red blood cells 24 hours after application. ×225. **d.** Skin graft capillary containing red blood cells 24 hours after application. ×300. **e.** Skin graft capillary that is grossly distended and packed with red blood cells 48 hours after application. ×200. Hynes (1954) Br. J. Plast. Surg. 6:257.

Summary

The phase of serum imbibition may be described as a period during which the graft vessels fill with a fibrinogen-free fluid and cells from the host bed. The term plasmatic circulation is actually a misnomer, because the fluid absorbed by the graft from the host bed is trapped within the graft. Endothelial ingrowth from the host progresses until a definitive vasculature is established. The stagnant fluid absorbed by the graft during the early phase of serum circulation is apparently drained off by the newly established blood and lymphatic circulation. Clinically, skin grafts in man usually appear edematous and their surfaces are elevated above the surrounding host skin during the early postoperative period. Within a few days after grafting, however, the graft flattens and edema subsides. This phenomenon reflects the establishment of plasmatic and hemic flow and the evacuation of the fluid initially trapped in the graft.

Phase of Graft Revascularization

Controversy has arisen over the method of graft acceptance and the mode of vascularization. Several research techniques have been developed to study the physiology of graft acceptance and vascularization. These techniques include gross and stereomicroscopic observations of the graft in situ, in vivo microscopy through transparent chambers and microangiography, histologic and histochemical analyses of skin biopsy specimens, and the injection of dyes or radioactive isotopes into the vascular system of the recipient animals. However, there is no ideal method of studying these processes in vivo; this limitation partially explains the persistent controversies surrounding the exact mode of revascularization.

Bert, in 1865, first noted an early connection between the blood vessels of the graft and host and employed the term "abouchement" (French for mouth-to-mouth contact) to illustrate the mouth-to-mouth apposition of the vessels. In 1874 Thiersch, studying the histologic sections of experimental full-thickness skin grafts in man, used the term "inosculation" to signify the direct connection between graft and host vessels.

Garré (1889), studying human skin grafts, reported evidence of endothelial mitosis in the host bed 5.5 hours after grafting, inflammatory cells in the grafts by 9 hours, and active invasion of wandering white cells into the donor vessels at 11 hours. He discounted the importance of the inosculatory process and described actual revascularization as an invasion of the graft by host capillary buds, which commenced on the third or fourth day, after most of the original vessels had become obliterated. Garré's conclusions agreed with those of Hübscher (1888), and a similar opinion was expressed by Goldmann (1890). Jungengel (1891) and Enderlen (1897) also maintained that most of the preexisting graft vessels degenerated, but some of the endothelial cells were able to survive and form new vessels that eventually connected with the ingrowing host vessels.

Braun (1899) was of the opinion that graft revascularization was achieved by a dual process of ingrowth of host vessels and anastomoses between the host and original graft vasculatures. Henle (1899), after injecting various dyes into rabbit recipients of full-thickness grafts, arrived at conclusions similar to those expressed by Garré, i.e., there is early evidence of endothelial mitosis followed by rapid capillary ingrowth from the recipient site: an extensive vascular network in the donor skin is reconstituted without the cooperation of the original graft vessels, which rapidly undergo degenerative changes. Henle felt that in time some of the invading host capillaries could penetrate and grow along the channels left by the necrosed graft vessels.

Most of the pioneer studies on the origin and development of the blood supply in skin grafts were experiments on split-thickness grafts performed during the years 1888–1897 (Hübscher 1888; Garré 1889; Goldmann 1890; Jungengel 1891; Enderlen 1897). There were many subsequent reports concerning the process of vascularization in transplanted skin, but no serious efforts were made to study the nature of vascularization in skin of varying thicknesses.

In 1925 Davis and Traut, employing intracardiac injections of China ink in dogs, observed that the anastomosis of graft and host vessels begins as early as 22 hours after application of the graft and persists for up to 72 hours (Fig. 6a and b). They also stressed subsequent host capillary growth (Fig. 6c), occurring by the fourth day, and concluded that it is the decisive factor involved in establishing the definitive vascular system of the graft. Mir y Mir (1951), experimenting with postmortem dye injection into the aorta, considered the thickness of skin grafts in dogs an important factor controlling the vascularization. According to Mir y Mir, the restoration of blood supply in the thin split-thickness skin graft is achieved mainly by the establishment of direct vascular continuity between the respective vessels of the graft and host. The sequence of vascular changes in full-thickness skin grafts as reported by Mir y Mir (1951) parallels that reported by Davis and Traut (1925): the vitality of such grafts is initially ensured by the direct vascular connections between the two tissues, followed, in turn, by extensive host vascular ingrowth. In his classic study, Medawar (1944) observed that the revascularization of skin grafts in the rabbit by the ingrowth of capillaries from the host bed is achieved 4 days after grafting (Fig. 7a); the original graft vessels, which he called "wound vessels," disappear between the fourth and eighth days after grafting (Fig. 7b).

Peer and Walker (1951) believed that the restoration of circulation in skin grafts is mainly achieved by direct connection between severed ends of blood vessels in the graft and host tissues and they stressed the importance of early vascular anastomosis for survival of the centrally located cells in the grafted tissue.

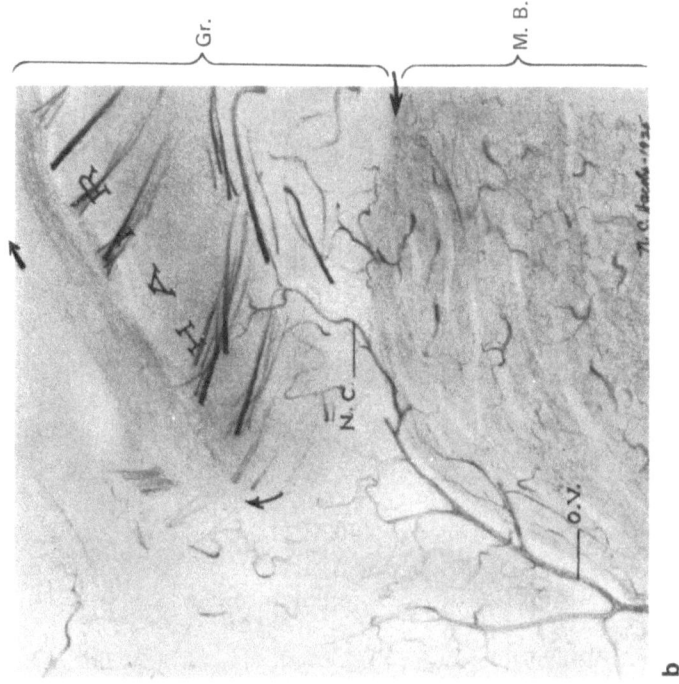

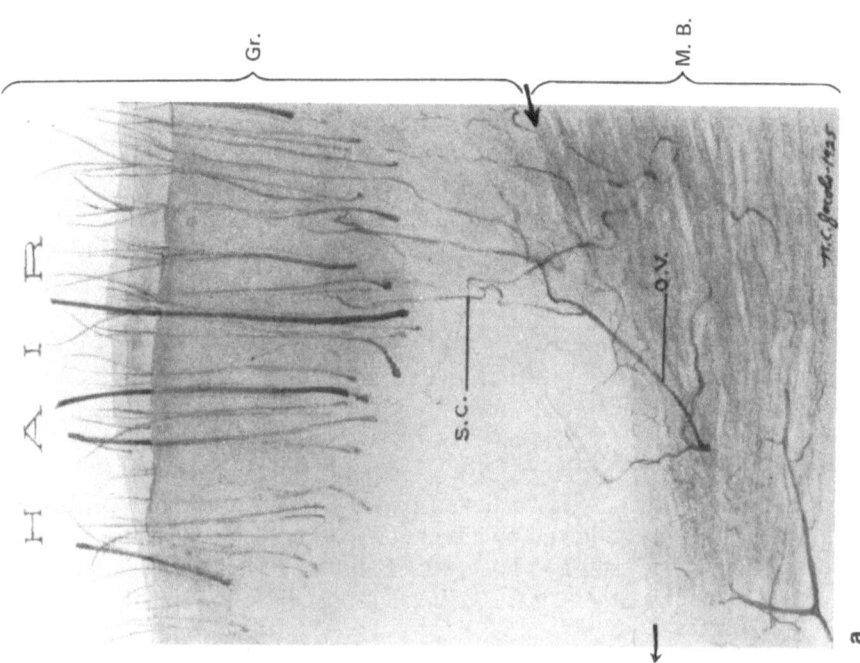

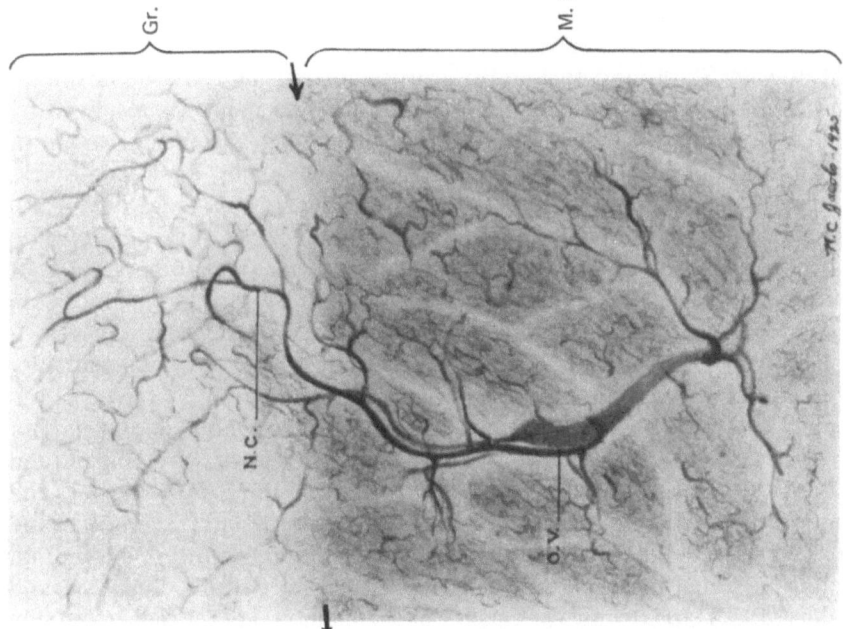

Fig. 6 a–c. Study of graft revascularization employing intracardiac injection of China ink in dogs. **a.** Injected and cleared specimen removed 3 days after operation. *Gr.*, full-thickness graft; *M.B.*, tissue on which graft was placed; *O.V.*, blood supply of the host tissue; *S.C.*, surviving capillaries; *arrows*, lower margins of the graft. The capillaries extend well up toward the surface of the skin and are quite extensive. These capillaries are injected at this early date because they have established anastomoses with the vessels of the host tissues.

b. Full-thickness graft with the superficial tissues closed over it. The specimen was removed 5 days after operation, injected, and cleared by the Spalteholtz method. The injected capillary in this specimen reaches upward to the tip of a papilla of the corium, i.e., to the malpighian layer. This is another example of the circulation of the graft being established by anastomosis. *Gr.*, full-thickness graft; *M.B.*, host tissue; *O.V.*, vessel of the host tissue; *N.C.*, capillary that has anastomosed with the underlying vessel; *arrows*, margin of the graft.

c. Specimen removed 41 days after operation. It was treated in a manner similar to those depicted in panels a and b. This is another mode of establishing the circulation of skin grafts. The capillary network of the graft is the result of upward growth from the host tissues. The plexus is extremely dense; later this becomes greatly modified, many of the vessels disappearing. *Gr.*, graft; *M.B.*, muscular host tissue; *O.V.*, vessel of the host tissue; *N.C.*, new capillaries; *arrows*, margin of the graft. Davis and Traut (1925) Ann. Surg. 82:871.

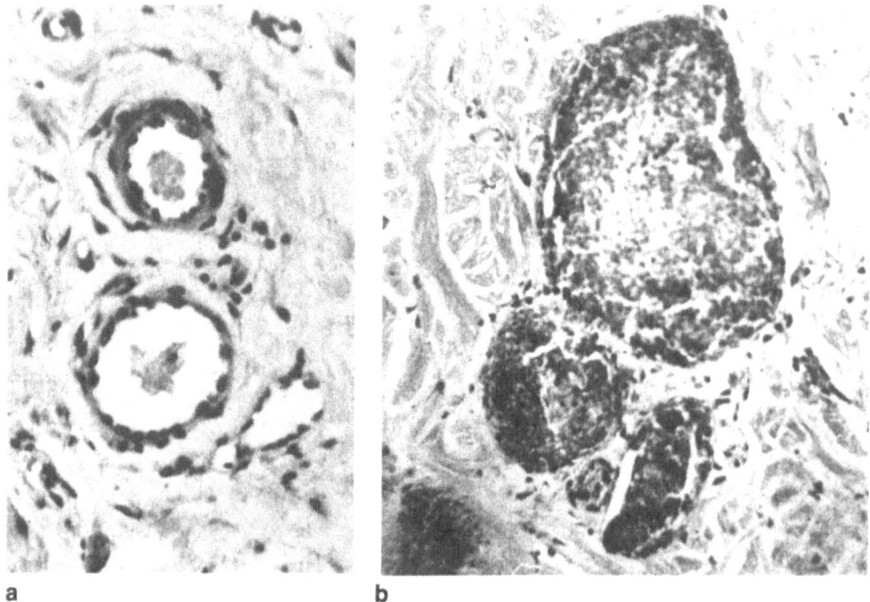

a   b

Fig. 7 a and b. Revasularization of skin graft in the rabbit. **a.** Differentiated vessels of the primary circulation in the lower reaches of the dermis of a 4-day allograft. The endothelial swelling is probably without specific significance. ×420. **b.** Stagnation of "wound vessels" in an 8-day allograft. Their endothelial lining has disappeared, and leukocytes arrested within the lumen of the vessel are pyknotic or otherwise degenerate. ×190. Medawar (1944) J. Anat. 78:176, Cambridge University Press.

Conway, Stark, and Joslin (1951), using a transparent tissue chamber, found that vascularization of skin *autografts* in the mouse is achieved by capillary budding in the host site and by subsequent vascular ingrowth of capillary sprouts into the grafts. In 1952 Conway, Joslin, Rees, and Stark, who used the same mouse chamber technique (Fig. 8a–c), and Ham (1952), who injected pigs with India ink suspension, stated that skin *allografts* do not become vascularized, offering this finding as an explanation of allograft rejection. However, Taylor and Lehrfeld (1953), by means of direct skin stereomicroscopy, observed that allografts in rats are successfully vascularized prior to the rejection reaction; their finding that autografts and allografts are both vascularized was confirmed in man by Converse and Rapaport (1956). These findings are consistent with histologic evidence of the vascularization of skin allografts in man, as reported by Gibson and Medawar (1943) and McGregor (1955 a,b). After injecting India ink and bromophenol blue into the circulatory system of rabbits, Scothorne and McGregor (1953) cited evidence of vascularization in allografts, but did not specify the actual process. Subsequently, Conway, Griffith, Shannon, and Findley (1957) and Conway, Sedar, and Shannon (1957), accepting the

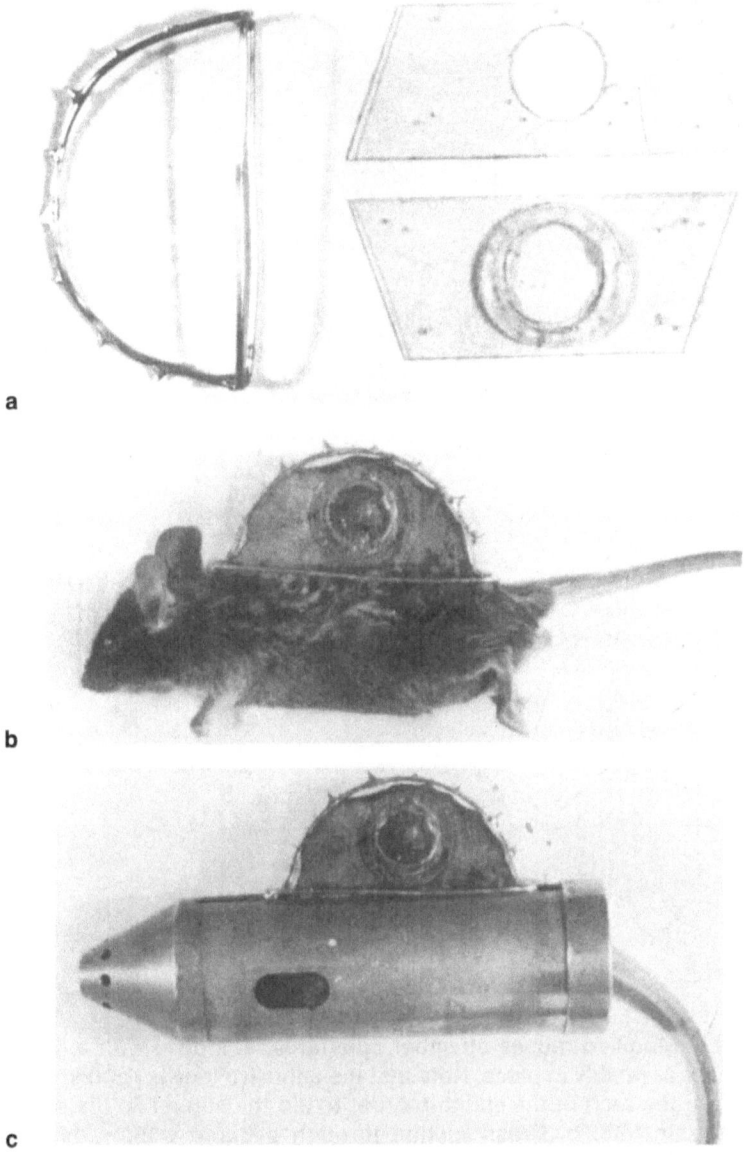

a

b

c

Fig. 8 a–c. Mouse chamber appartus for in vivo microscopic study of revas-cularization. **a.** Traction splint of copper wire which acts as an immobilization framework. A mated pair of lucite splints, one of which contains the tissue chamber, is incorporated into the immobilization device by the use of through-and-through sutures of tantalum wire. **b.** Joslin's modified transparent tissue chamber in place upon the dorsum of a mouse. **c.** Metal cartridge holder. The vent allows the tissue chamber to be viewed directly under the microscope. Conway, Joslin, Rees, and Stark (1952) Plast. Reconstr. Surg. 9:557, © (1952) The Williams & Wilkins Co., Baltimore.

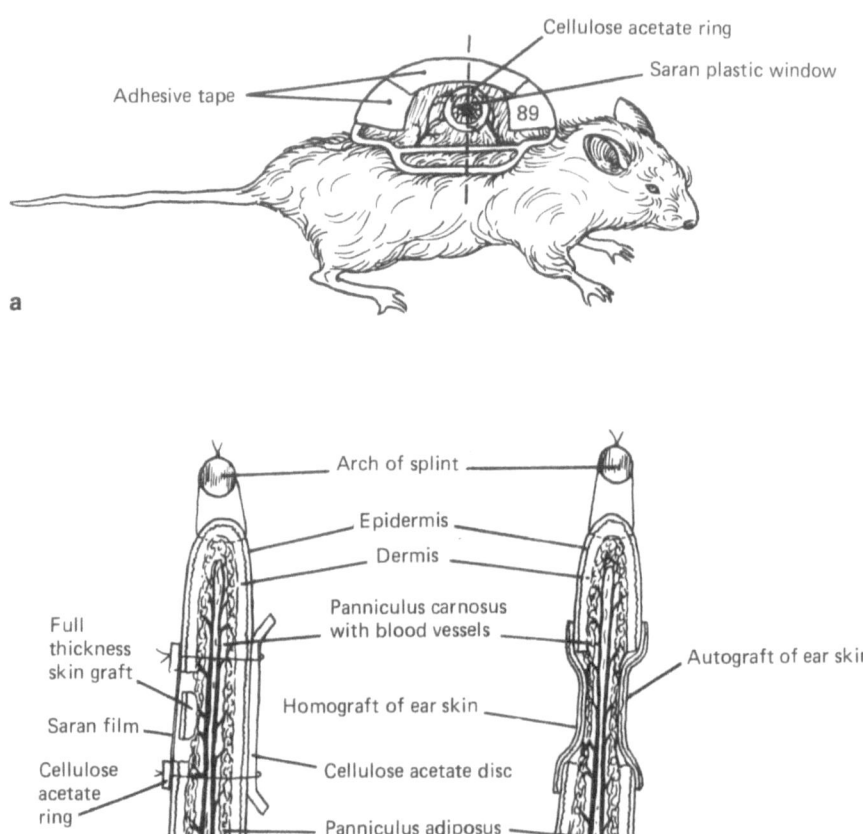

Fig. 9 a–c. Modified mouse chamber apparatus. **a.** Mouse with a new splint and chamber assembly in place. Note that the adhesive tape is applied along the full length of the arch of the splint in order to aid the sutures in the support of the dorsal skin fold. **b.** Cross section through a Saran window preparation placed at the level of the vertical broken line in part a. A full-thickness graft of the skin of the middorsum is covered by the thin film of Saran plastic. Note that the graft is not fitted to the edges of the recipient bed and that it is much thicker than the full-thickness grafts of the skin of the ear shown in part c. **c.** Cross section through a "natural" window preparation placed at the level of the vertical broken line in part a. The full-thickness grafts of the skin of the ear are applied on both sides of the dorsal skin fold. Note the simplicity of this arrangement. Conway, Griffith, Shannon, and Findley (1957) Plast. Reconstr. Surg. 20:103, © (1957) The Williams & Wilkins Co., Baltimore.

criticisms of Scothorne and McGregor (1953) and Taylor and Lehrfeld (1953), modified their transparent apparatus (Fig. 9) and reported evidence of active blood circulation in murine skin allografts.

Stereomicroscopic Studies

The technique of observing cutaneous blood vessels in skin in vivo was described by Lombard in 1911–1912 and developed by Lewis in 1927. The stereomicroscopic technique developed by Taylor and Lehrfeld (1953, 1955) for the direct observation of the vascularization in rat skin grafts (Fig. 10) was modified for experimental studies in man (Fig. 11) by Converse and Rapaport (1956). The stereomicroscopic appearance of autografts and allografts has been fully described, with particular attention to vascular changes, by Taylor and Lehrfeld (1953, 1955) in the rat (Fig. 12) and by Converse and Rapaport (1956) in man (Fig. 13). These changes may be summarized as follows: immediately after application to the recipient bed and during the subsequent 24 hours, the blood vessels of the graft appear less filled with blood and are not readily detected when compared with those in the surrounding skin. On the first day after grafting, many vessels in the donor tissue show early evidence of distention and are rapidly filled with static blood (Fig. 12b). On the second day vessel distention continues, but blood circulation has not commenced (Figs. 12c and 13a), although a sluggish flow of blood may occasionally be seen in the peripheral vessels. A slow flow of

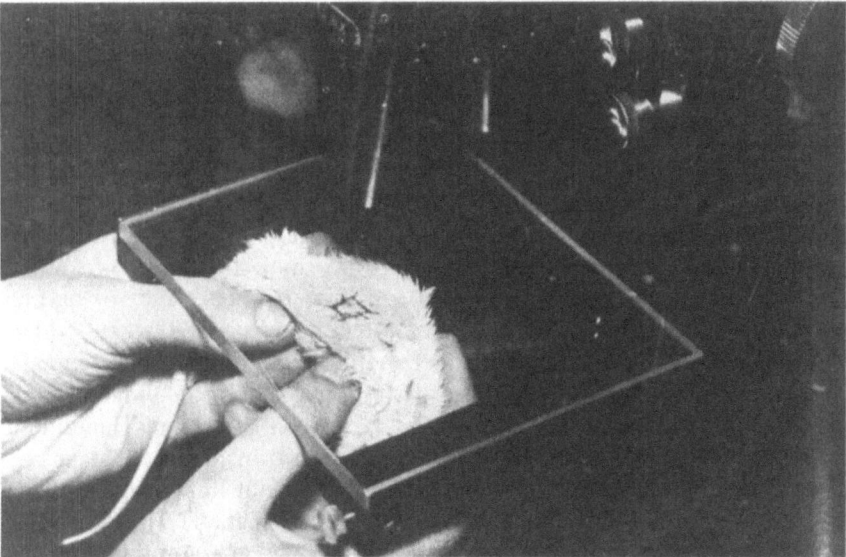

Fig. 10. Manner of holding animal to study skin graft by stereomicroscopic technique. Taylor and Lehrfeld (1955) Ann. N.Y. Acad. Sci. 59:351.

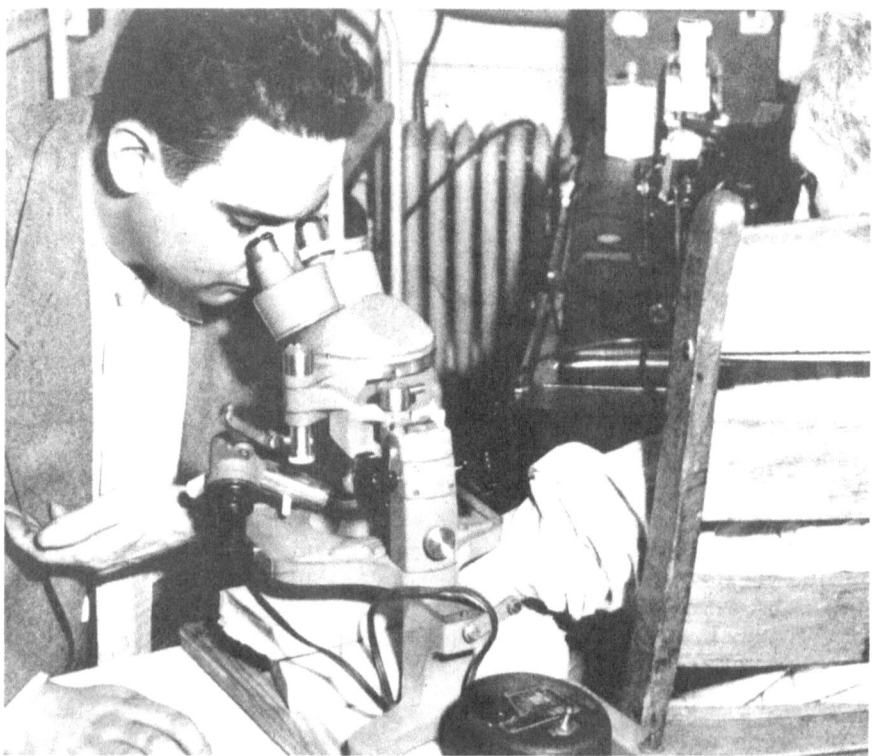

Fig. 11. Stereomicroscope employed for direct observation of skin graft vessels in man. Converse and Rapaport (1956) Ann. Surg. 143:306.

blood occurs in the graft vasculature on the third or fourth day (Figs. 12d and e and 13b) and continues to improve until the fifth or sixth day (Fig. 13c). During the subsequent days, a return of all blood vessels to normal caliber and circulation generally occurs in all autografts.

In allografts, the similarity persists only until the onset of allograft rejection. As reviewed in more detail in Chapter 2 (see pages 61 and 65), rejection is heralded by increased distention in the vascular system, followed by sluggish circulation with clumped elements (Figs. 12f and 13d). Complete cessation of blood flow and vascular disruption in most skin allografts (Figs. 12g and h and 13e and f) usually occur 7–10 days after transplantation.

The direct observation of the vessels in skin transplants by means of a dissecting microscope, as practiced by Converse and Rapaport (1956), has also been used by Ceppellini, Curtoni, Mattiuz, Leigheb, Visetti, and Columbi (1966) for assessing vascularization and survival end points of human skin grafts. Although the use of skin stereomicroscopy is a useful tool for determining changes in the appearance and state of blood circulation in the

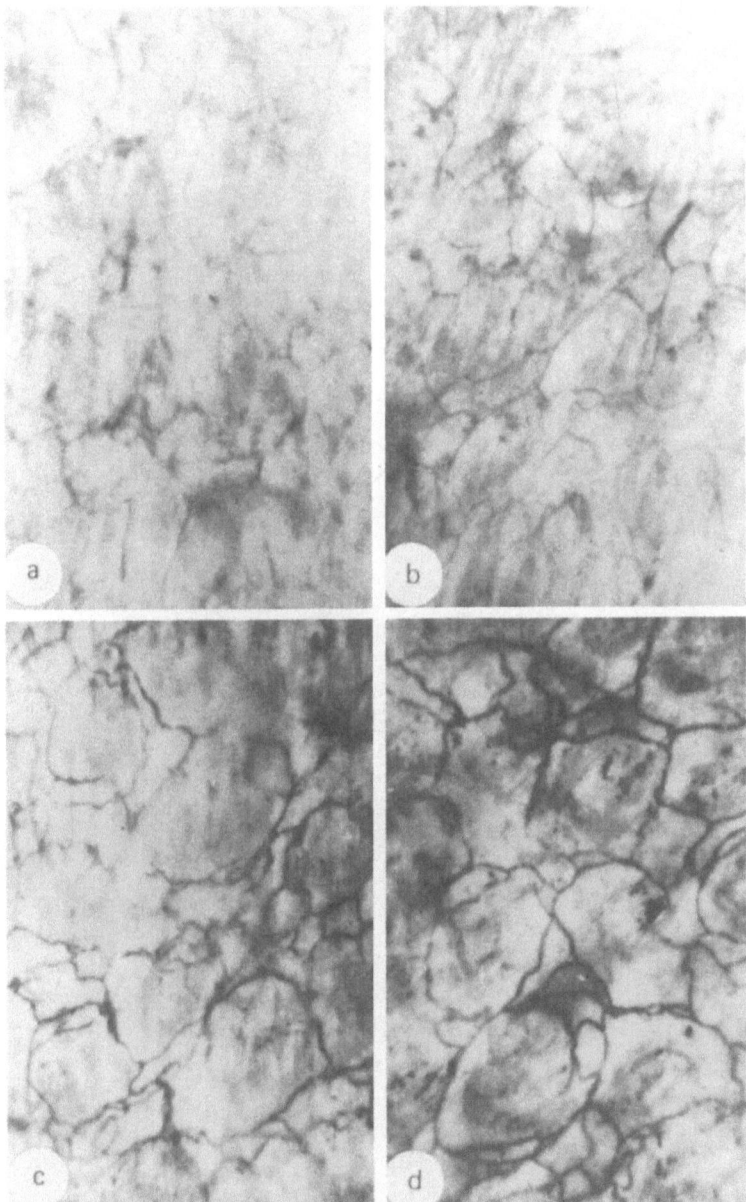

Fig. 12 a–h. Stereomicrographic appearance of minute vessels of rat allograft.
a. Normal intact rat skin. **b.** Allograft 1 day after transplantation shows some
distention of the vessels, indicating partial filling with blood. **c.** After 2 days more
vessels are distended with blood but there is no flow. **d.** After 3 days there is
considerable distention of all vessels but little movement of contained blood.

(Continued on page 20)

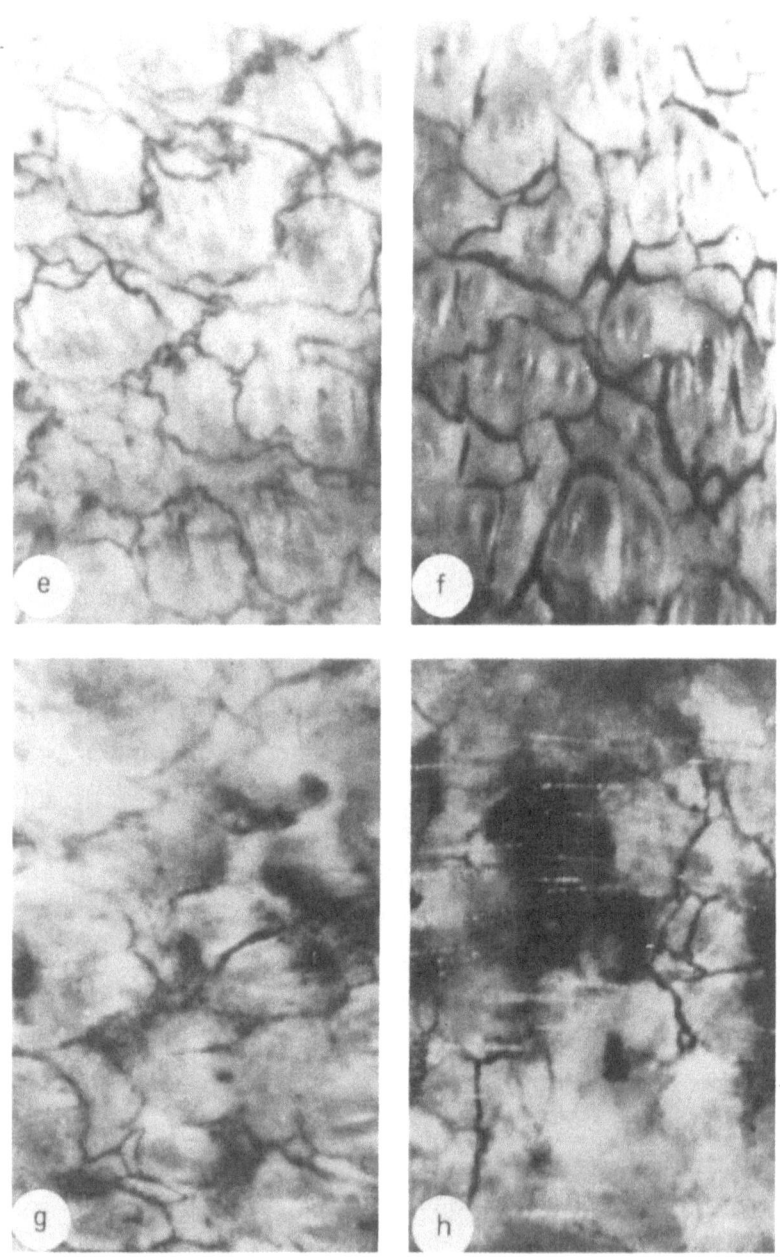

(Figure 12 continued)
e. Circulation, though slow, is visible in all vessels after 4 days. **f.** By 8 days after transplantation the distention of all vessels and a generalized stasis of blood indicate the beginning of the rejection reaction. **g and h.** After 9 days vascular breakdown is characterized by local hemorrhage, first apparent around smaller capillary loops and then involving the larger vessels. Taylor and Lehrfeld (1955) Ann. N.Y. Acad. Sci. 59:351.

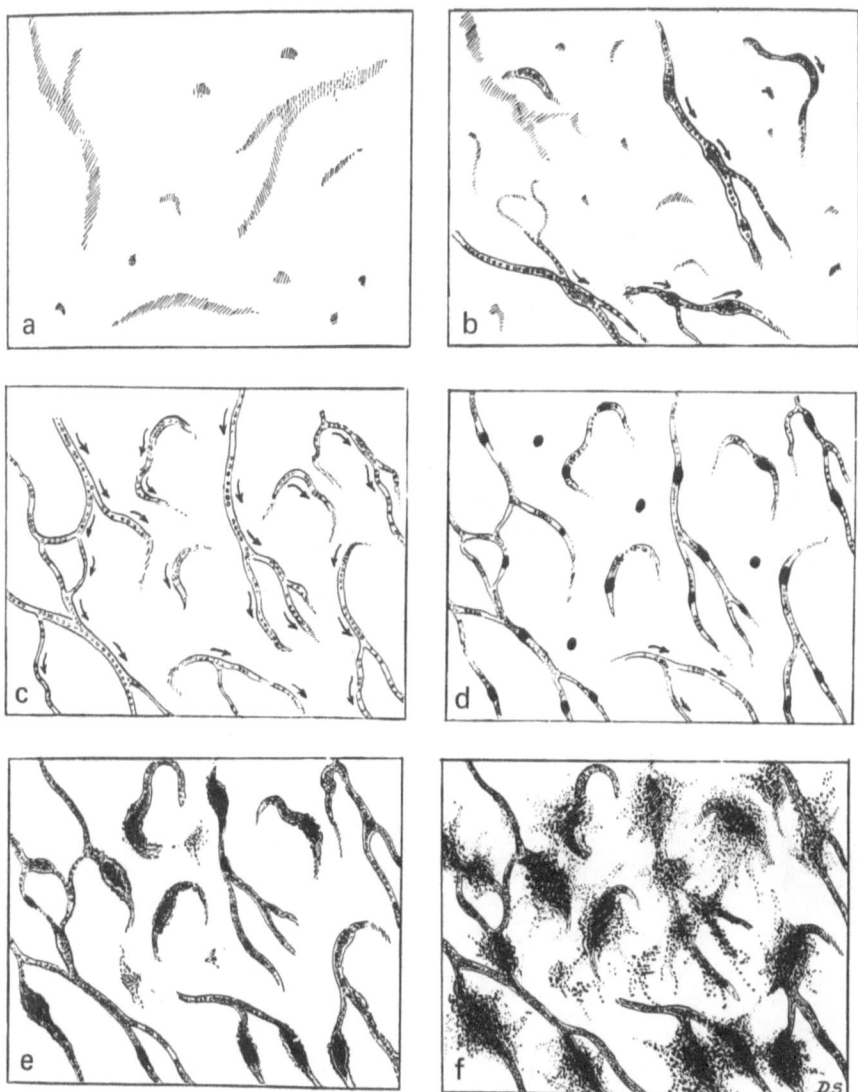

Fig. 13 a–f. Stereomicroscopic appearance of minute vessels of human skin grafts. **a.** Dilated vessels can first be seen 48 hours after transplantation. **b.** On the third or fourth day a sluggish flow is established. **c.** Active flow is observed by the fifth or sixth day. **d.** Multiple thrombi appear in the vessels of the allografts around the eighth day and flow ceases. **e.** In allografts the thrombosed vessels are dilated during the subsequent 20 hours. **f.** The final event in all allografts is the rupture of the vessel walls with extravasation of blood rendering further stereomicroscopic examination impossible. Converse and Rapaport (1956) Ann. Surg. 143:306.

grafted tissue from the time of transplantation to the appearance of the rejection reaction, this direct method is not adequate for defining the actual source of vascular supply and the mode of vascularization in various types of skin grafts.

Histologic Studies

Henry, Marshall, Friedman, Goldstein, and Dammin (1961) and Henry, Marshall, Friedman, Dammin, and Merrill (1962), following their histologic studies in humans, attributed the vascularization of auto- and allografts of skin to the inosculation of the patent original capillaries in the deeper layers of the graft dermis with the capillary loops from the host bed. As a consequence of even a few initial vascular connections, the superficial graft capillaries, whose endothelial linings had degenerated during the first few days after transplantation, are supplied with blood and become dilated. The authors infer that this feature persists until the superficial channels are reconstituted by endothelial cells growing along the existing vessels. Their histologic study showed no vascular connections between the donor and host skin for 2 days following transplantation; during this time, the superficial capillaries in the graft collapse and the endothelial cells degenerate, leaving the basement membrane intact (Fig. 14). Although the graft vascular system appears dilated and engorged with static blood by the second or third day, the superficial vessels continue to demonstrate an intact basement

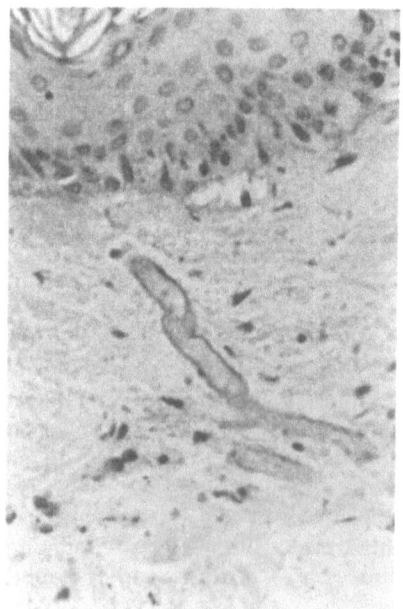

Fig. 14.   Histology of first-set allograft in man, day 2. The epidermis shows early degenerative changes but the epidermal basement membrane is intact. The endothelial cells of the capillary in the upper dermis have disappeared but the capillary basement membrane is still present. PAS. ×350. Henry, Marshall, Friedman, Dammin, and Merrill (1962) J. Clin. Invest. 41:420.

membrane with the endothelial nuclei either pyknotic or entirely absent; in the meantime the original vessels located in the deep dermal layers of the graft appear patent on histologic examination. The process of graft vascularization is completed on the sixth or seventh day, as histologically evidenced by patent capillaries in the deep layers of the dermis and distended superficial capillaries.

Other Experimental Studies

A modification of the Algire transparent chamber was developed by Edgerton and Edgerton (1955) to evaluate the vascular activity of mouse skin grafts. Their findings are somewhat similar to those recorded by Taylor and Lehrfeld (1953) and Converse and Rapaport (1956). In the chamber, Edgerton and Edgerton noted vigorous vascular ingrowth from the host into the graft filling the original graft vascular system with static blood as early as the second and third day. Subsequently, flow velocity, which is sluggish soon after the establishment of some vascular connections between the host and graft, progressively increases to a normal rate after the third or fourth day after grafting. They concluded that the vascular continuity between the original graft vessels and host vessels plays an important role in the establishment of a definitive vasculature with active hemic circulation in the graft. A similar opinion was expressed by Kamrin (1960, 1961), who held that in rat auto- and allografts the ingrowth of capillary buds from the recipient site has achieved contact with the original graft vessels by the end of the fourth day or the beginning of the fifth day, as shown on histologic examination by the sudden emptying of the crenated (deformed) erythrocytes from the clotted graft vascular system and the subsequent replacement by normal host blood elements.

In a previous study by Egdahl, Good, and Varco (1957), attention was called to the disappearance of intradermally injected fluorescein during the early stages of vascularization in 50 full-thickness rat allografts. These workers noted the disappearance of intradermal fluorescein as early as 12 hours prior to the onset of blood circulation, as shown by the direct skin stereomicroscopic method of Taylor and Lehrfeld (1953). "The removal of fluorescein test" and the capacity to develop a localized Schwartzman phenomenon[1] in first-set allografts are considered to be strong evidence of successful vascularization via direct connections between vessels of the graft and those of the recipient. Castermans (1957), who applied vital microscopic methods to skin autografts and allografts in mice, obtained somewhat similar results. According to Castermans, the graft capillaries commence to

---

[1] Schwartzman phenomenon: a form of focal reaction characterized by a hemorrhagic and necrotic skin lesion in specifically hypersensitive rabbits following intradermal injections of homologous or heterologous bacterial antigens.

fill with formed hemic elements and dilate as early as 24 hours after grafting, followed by initial blood flow at 48 hours; at day 6 or 7 the capillary network is well developed and functional, although still distended.

In an attempt to evaluate the source of blood supply in the autologous and allogeneic transplants of mouse and rat skin, Rolle, Taylor, and Charipper (1959) utilized a combination of the following four methods of examination: direct skin microscopy, routine histologic methods, cardiac injections of India ink suspensions into the vascular system, and intravenous injections of a diffusible dye, bromophenol blue. They found that many of the graft vessels, empty at the time of removal from the donor, commence to acquire stagnant blood and appear distended by 24 hours after surgery. At 3 days, the blood circulation within the graft vasculature is restored and resumes the normal velocity of blood flow the following day; there is no histologic evidence of degenerative changes in the original graft vessels. Rolle and her co-workers (1959), as well as Hildemann and Haas (1960), concluded that the definitive vasculature in the graft capable of supporting an active circulation appears to depend on the direct vascular continuity between the host and graft, not the newly formed vessels from the host.

Ljungqvist and Almgård (1966) used a combined stereomicroangio-graphic (Fig. 15a) and histologic method (Fig. 15b) at varying time intervals after transplantation to determine the vascular changes in skin auto- and allografts on the auricles of rabbits. The results indicated that the ingrowth of precapillary and capillary vessels from the underlying host bed, first noted 2 days after operation, invades the graft and extends in a perpendicular and spiral fashion toward the dermoepidermal surface, replacing the degenerated graft vessels. These ingrowing vessels form the definitive vasculature of the graft. While there is some evidence of direct connection between the graft and host blood systems, the degenerative changes with thrombosis in the preexisting graft vessels suggest that these vascular connections play a minor and temporary role.

In 1974 Guthy, Billote, and Burke used daily gross and in vivo stereomicroscopic observations, coupled with histopathologic examination of skin biopsy specimens, to determine the sequence of events in full-thickness skin auto- and allografts in the guinea pig. Their data, collected on the fourth day after operation, indicate minimal granulation tissue in the bed, good graft–host coaptation, and excellent graft vascularization, as demonstrated by a pink color, blanching and refilling upon the application of digital pressure. These findings appear to corroborate the histologic findings that numerous vascular buds originate from venules and precapillary arterioles in the recipient site and form direct vascular continuity with preexisting graft vessels via temporary thin-walled vascular lakes, presumably of graft origin. At this time, the original graft and invading host vessels are engorged with red blood cells. Consequently, the authors considered that the ingrowing host vessels and subsequent anastomoses with the original graft vessels play an important role in the establishment of the definitive skin graft vasculature.

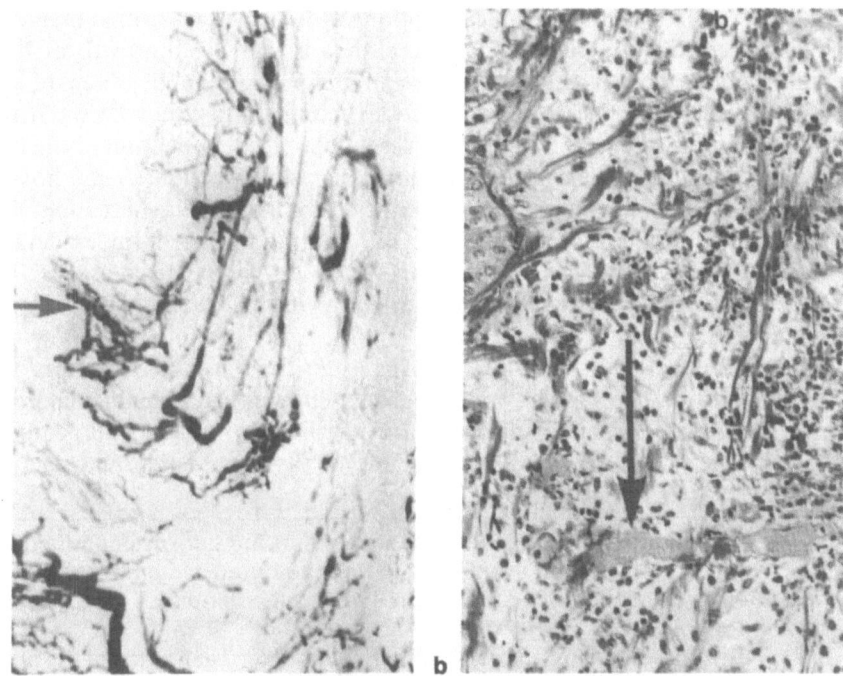

Fig. 15 a and b. Combined stereomicroangiographic and histologic study of rabbit auricle allograft. **a.** Microangiogram including the graft–host junction *(arrow)* of an allograft 4 days after transplantation. *Above arrow:* host tissue is vascularized by a regular network of mainly delicate vessels. *Below arrow:* graft is vascularized by irregularly coursing vessels of varying calibers, most evident in lower left corner of picture. ×25. **b.** Histologic section from the area depicted in panel a. The graft is edematous and infiltrated by mononuclear and some polymorphonuclear cells. *Arrow:* a contrast-filled vessel. Van Gieson–elastic. ×135. Ljungqvist and Almgård (1966) Acta Pathol. Microbiol. Scand. 68:553.

Histochemical Studies

In the past, relatively few histochemical methods had been employed to evaluate the metabolic changes occurring in skin transplants (Scothorne and Tough 1952; Scothorne and Scothorne 1953; Thompson 1962; Russell and Monaco 1965); no efforts were made to define the phase of graft vascularization. In order to study this problem under experimental conditions that more closely approximated the events occurring in orthotopic grafting, autografts and allografts placed on mammalian recipients were studied by Converse and Ballantyne (1962) by means of an enzyme histochemical method.

The reagents employed, neotetrazolium chloride and reduced diphosphopyridine nucleotide (DPNH), indicate the presence of DPNH dehydrogenase (DPN diaphorase) in the fresh frozen sections (Antopol, Glaubach, and Goldman 1950). Histochemical sections of full-thickness skin autografts and allografts in rats (Fig. 16a–e) have shown that the ingrowth of host capillaries into skin transplants is essential for the establishment of the definitive vasculature of the graft. The structural differences between the preexisting graft and new blood host vessels permit identification of the two types of vasculature. The process of graft revascularization by the host is very rapid; the host capillaries penetrate through the demarcation line into the graft dermis by 6 hours (Fig. 16a) and attain the dermoepidermal junction by 48 hours. The data in this study also indicate a progressive decline of enzymatic activity, accompanied by degenerative changes, in the original graft vasculature during the first 4 days after grafting. In contrast to the vasculature of the surrounding host tissue, the vascular pattern in the graft is changed. The vessels are numerous, show greater ramification and distention (Fig. 16b), and a purposeful and parallel ingrowth in a perpendicular direction from the recipient bed (Fig. 16c) to the dermoepidermal junction

Fig. 16 a–h. (Opposite). Histochemical sections of full-thickness grafts demonstrating course of vascular events. **a.** Six-hour autograft. Note the host blood capillaries that have penetrated the union line into the dermis of the autograft. ×110.

b. Twenty-four-hour autograft. The epidermal and dermal tissues of the autograft *(right)* and host *(left)* are intimately united. The blood vessels in the host bed show increased distention and endothelial activity. ×32.

c. Two-day autograft. Note new host capillary originating from the distended vessel in the recipient bed and growing perpendicular to the graft. The new vessel is wavy in contour with thin endothelial lining; the vessel from which the host vessel originated is cylindrical and straight with thick endothelial lining. ×225.

d. Three-day autograft. The graft dermis is revascularized by the host vessels. Note the parallel ingrowth of numerous distended host vessels into the graft dermis. ×40.

e. Four-day allograft. The allograft is completely revascularized by parallel ingrowth of numerous branched host vessels. ×40.

f. Eight-day allograft. Note the complete loss of DPN diaphorase activity in the allograft vessels during the rejection period. Pilosebaceous structures and epidermis show an advanced loss of enzymatic activity. ×45.

g. Seven-day allograft. The early disappearance of diaphorase activity in the graft blood vessels begin a few hours prior to the cessation of blood flow. Complete loss of enzymatic activity of the vessels the following day is shown in panel h. ×40.

h. Eight-day allograft. Graft blood vessels at this time are no longer visible. Panels g and h are representative of the histochemical appearance of two of the five grafts, which were taken from a donor and transplanted concurrently to a single recipient on the seventh and eighth postoperative days, respectively. ×80. Converse and Ballantyne (1962) Plast. Reconstr. Surg. 30:415, © (1962) The Williams & Wilkins Co., Baltimore.

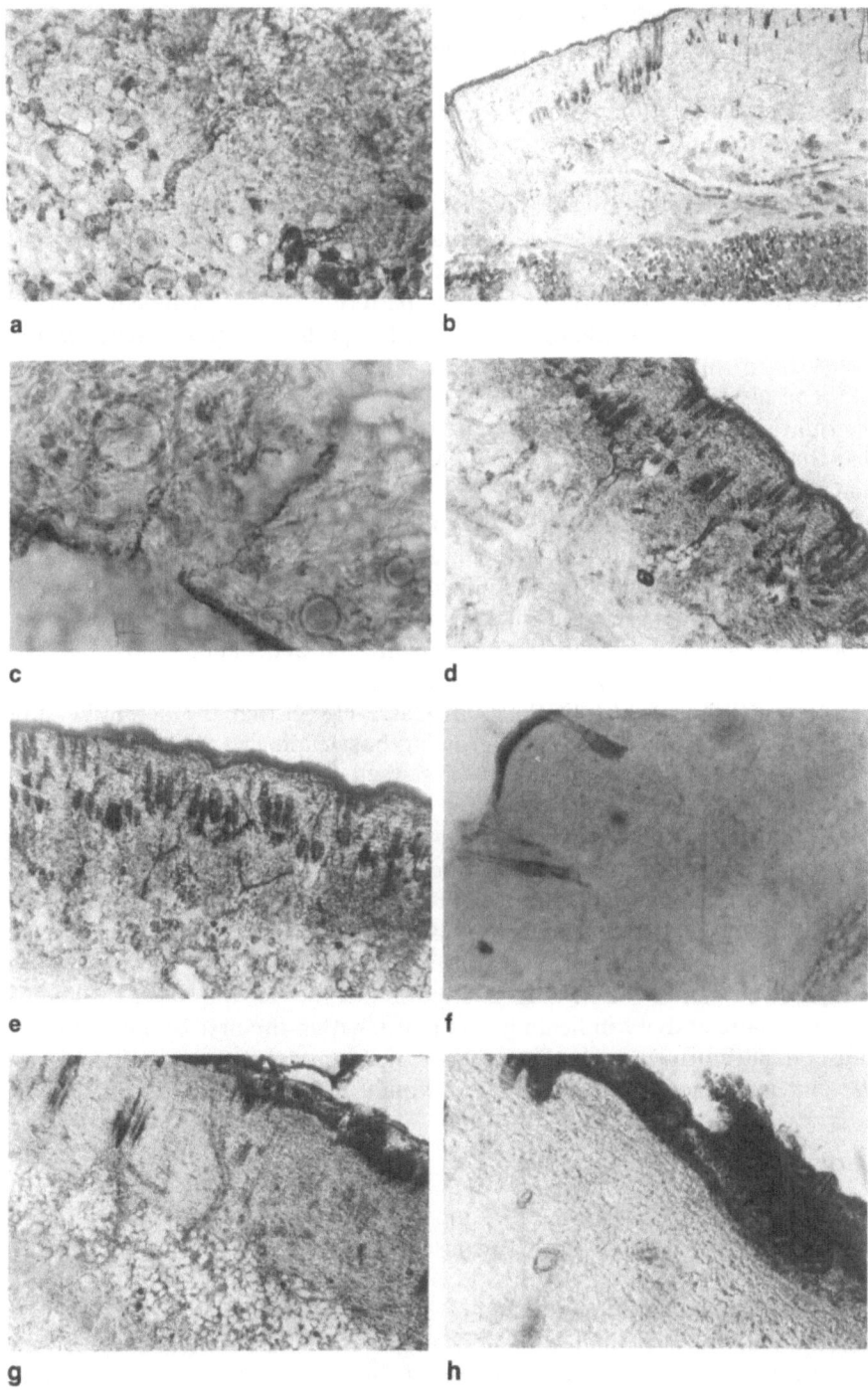

of the graft (Fig. 16d). The new vasculature progressively returns to a finer pattern during the following days. These findings appear to corroborate the stereomicroscopic observations of a progressive distention of the vessels and an increase in their number during the first few days after grafting (Taylor and Lehrfeld 1953; Converse and Rapaport 1956; Ballantyne and Converse 1957). The dilated vessels resume a fine caliber and become less numerous during the ensuing days. For the first 6 days after operation, the vascular changes associated with revascularization by the host in the full-thickness skin autografts and allografts are similar. However, during the following days the extent of the vascular pattern in allografts depends largely upon the occurrence of changes associated with the rejection reaction of the skin.

The histochemical studies of Converse and Ballantyne (1962) showed the rapid vascular ingrowth from the host into the graft, strongly suggesting that the new vessels are capable of establishing an adequate blood circulation in the graft within a short time. Although these findings established beyond a doubt that an actual ingrowth of new vessels from the host occurs, it could not be inferred that inosculation does not take place.

Subsequent histochemical studies using various hydrolytic and oxidative enzymes in porcine split-thickness skin grafts (see the section on Split-Thickness Grafts) were conducted by Wolff and Schellander (1965, 1966a). They confirmed the enzymatic observations of Converse and Ballantyne (1962) and the original hypothesis of Garré (1889) that the definitive skin graft vasculature is formed by ingrowing host capillaries (Fig. 17).

A divergent view suggested by Pedersen, Matthiessen, and Garbarsch (1970), working with skin autografts in the rat, is that the histochemical methods of assessment used by Converse and Ballantyne (1962), Converse, Filler, and Ballantyne (1965) (see the section on Split-Thickness Grafts), and Wolff and Schellander (1965) are not reliable criteria of graft viability. This opinion is based on observations indicating a more distinct and intense enzymatic activity in grafts and skin from dead rats during the first 3 days compared to that of the healing skin grafts. Moreover, the initial decline of the enzymatic activity in healing skin grafts within the first 24 hours and its subsequent return suggests the presence of a factor that temporarily inhibits the enzymatic activity at the time of wound healing.

Early Filling of the Vessels

Haller and Billingham (1964, 1967) and Haller et al. (1966) studied the origin of the vasculature in skin grafts using the cheek pouch of Syrian hamsters (Fig. 18a and b). Since it is devoid of pigmentation and appendages, the skinlike tissue constituting the highly vascular cheek pouch is almost transparent. When transplanted to genetically compatible hosts, it offers a window through which serial observation of the developing circulation can be

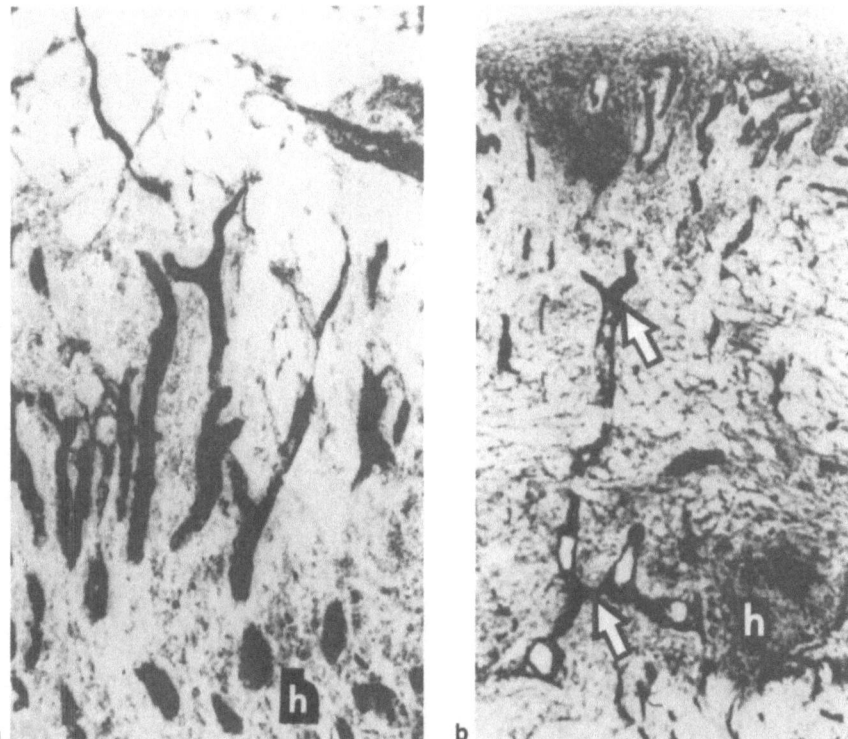

Fig. 17 a and b. Histochemical sections of porcine split-thickness skin grafts studied with ATPase method. **a.** After 5 days, strong enzymatic activity is observed in vessels invading the graft after having crossed the healing zone *(h)*. ×23. **b.** After 12 days, a highly positive vessel *(arrows)* originating from the healing zone *(h)* is penetrating the dermis of the graft. ×47. Wolff and Schellander (1966) J. Invest. Dermatol. 46:205. © (1966) The Williams & Wilkins Co., Baltimore.

made. The authors reported that following transplantation the blood vessels filled immediately, but no flow was noted before the fourth or fifth day; the patterns of blood vessels in the healed isografts were identical to those of the original graft vessels (Fig. 18c). The authors noted (1966, 1967) that when these vessels were blocked by previous injections of silicone rubber the grafts became necrotic, strongly suggesting that the intrinsic vessels of the graft are utilized for its survival.

Revascularization from the Host Bed Margins

Rees, Ballantyne, Hawthorne, and Nathan (1968) inserted silicone rubber sheeting between a suprapannicular skin autograft and the host bed in rats.

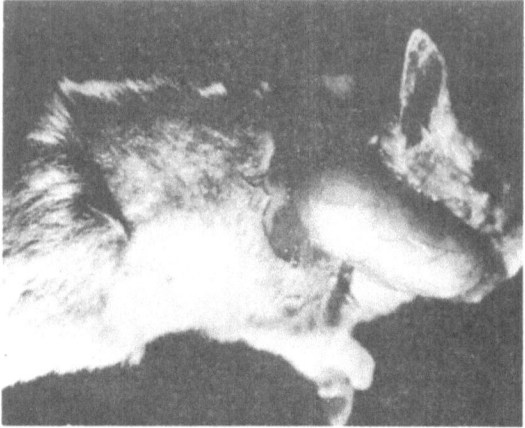

a

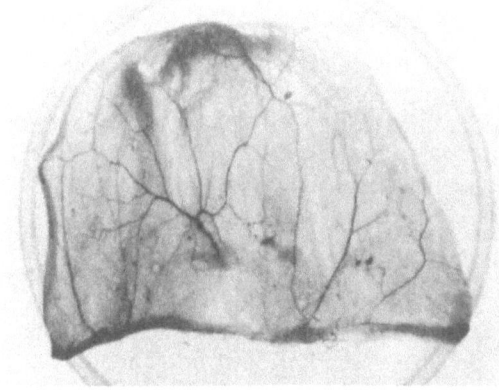

b

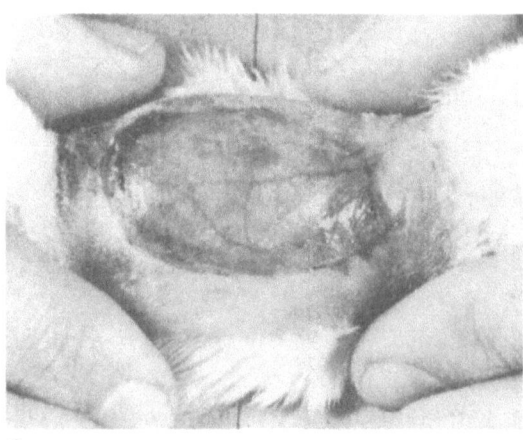

c

Fig. 18 a–c. Study of revascularization of skin graft in cheek pouch of Syrian hamster. **a.** Hamster's cheek pouch exposed by removal of the overlying integument. This structure has been filled with absorbent cotton. Note the prominent vasculature in its transparent wall. **b.** Excised cheek pouch opened to produce a more or less flat sheet of pouch skin. The vascular pattern is clearly visible. **c.** Pouch skin graft 14 days after transplantation. The orientation of its original vessels was in the long axis of the host's body. The original pattern has been faithfully maintained. Haller and Billingham (1964) in: Montagna and Billingham (eds.) Advances in Biology of Skin, vol. 5, MacMillan, N.Y.

The insertion of the silicone rubber sheets failed to prevent the development of a blood supply in these small skin grafts. This finding strongly supports the concept that, while vessels in the host bed may well be the main source of graft revascularization, the ingrowth of new vessels from the margins of the host bed can also play an important role in the vascularization of skin transplants. The success of revascularization of the graft from the margins of the host bed is inversely proportional to the size of the graft.

Studies in Microcirculation

A modification of the mouse skin transparent chamber of Merwin and Algire (1956) was used by Zarem, Zweifach, and McGehee (1967) to evaluate the development of microcirculation in full-thickness skin autografts in mice. Their microscopic findings indicate that endothelial budding arises from the small arteries and veins in the host bed rather than from capillaries or arterioles and venules. The endothelial buds then progress along the original graft vessels, which serve as nonviable conduits, and develop into an immature plexus of thin-walled, irregular channels with an oscillatory or slow unidirectional flow. By the eighth day after transplantation the immature plexus differentiates into arterioles, capillaries, and venules. Based on their observations, the authors believe that the reestablishment of the graft vasculature occurs primarily as a vascular ingrowth from the host.

In a subsequent experiment, O'Donoghue and Zarem (1971), using the same chamber technique in mice, evaluated the differences in the angiogenic properties of fresh skin isografts, fresh skin allografts, lyophilized isografts, and frozen–thawed isografts. It was reported that despite a consistent difference in the angiogenic properties of the various types of grafts, all grafts are capable of inducing hyperemia in the host beds (Fig. 19a) and neovascularization, consisting of the formation of host vascular buds and the development of sausage-shaped vessels extending toward the graft (Fig. 19b); all grafts are effectively vascularized (Fig. 19c). In both the fresh iso- and allografts, hyperemia is apparent on the third or fourth day after transplantation, neovascularization by the sixth day, and complete graft revascularization by the eighth day (the studies concerning the fate of preserved grafts are reviewed in Chapter 6). The authors concluded that the original graft vasculature plays an important role in stimulating the vascular budding from the host site, either to anastomose with the graft vessels or to penetrate the entire graft tissue.

Birch and Brånemark (1969) placed a full-thickness scrotal skin autograft over a thin vascular bed of outer auricular perichondrium and used the modified ear chamber (Fig. 3) of Brånemark and Lindström (1963) for vital microscopic evaluation in the rabbit (Fig. 20). Immediately after surgery, the authors observed filling of most graft vessels with partially hemolyzed blood (Fig. 20a). Sometimes because of the pumping effect of normal ear pulsa-

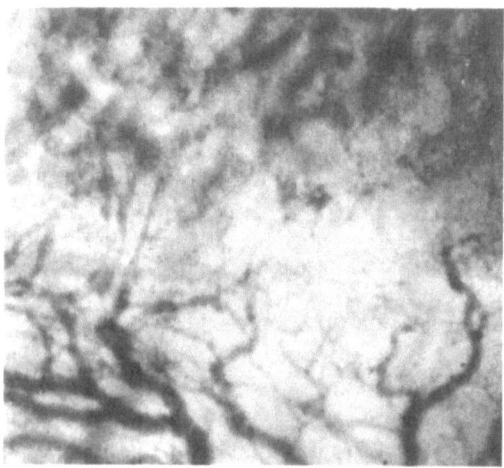

a

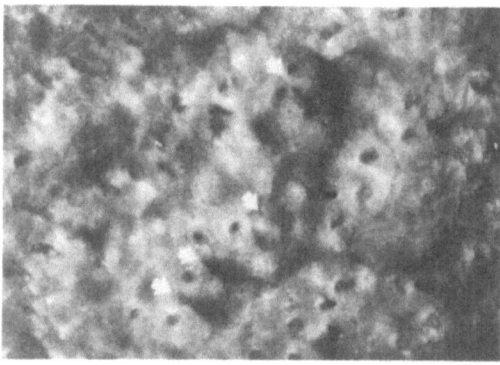

b

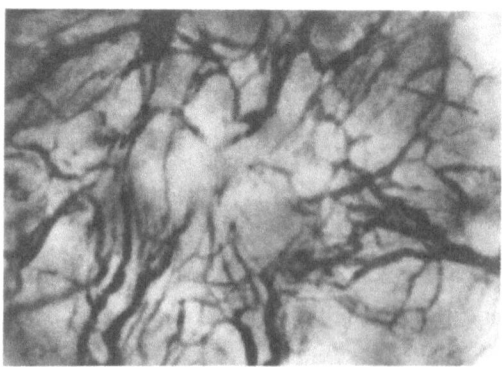

c

Fig. 19 a–c. Development of microcirculation in grafts in the mouse. **a.** The underlying tissue vessels *(lower half of photomicrograph)* are dilated 3 days after transplantation. ×210. **b.** Vascular buds *(arrows)* can be seen through a full-thickness skin graft 4 days after transplantation. ×200. **c.** Early vascularization of a full-thickness skin graft is apparent 6 days after transplantation. ×200. O'Donoghue and Zarem (1971) Plast. Reconstr. Surg. 48:474, © (1971) The Williams & Wilkins Co., Baltimore.

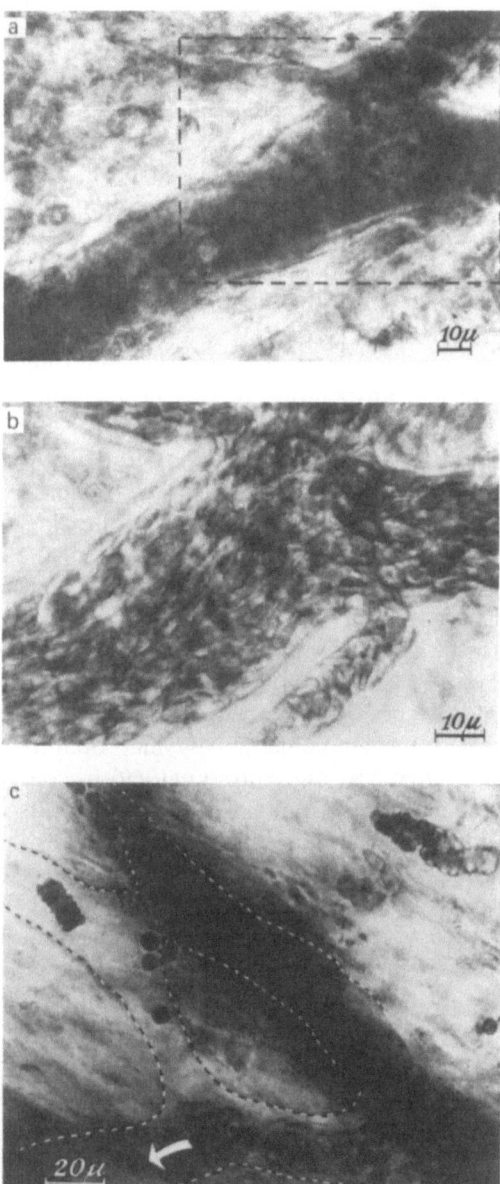

Fig. 20 a–c. Vital photomicrographs of scrotal skin autograft to rabbit's ear. **a.** Stationary hemolyzed blood is seen in autograft immediately after grafting. *Broken rectangle:* outline of the area shown in panel b. **b.** After 48 hours rapidly circulating erythrocytes fill the vessel. **c.** After 72 hours thin-walled proliferating vascular channels contain erythrocytes that exhibit slight to and fro movements with each heart beat. These vessels are seen at the extreme periphery of the graft. *Broken line:* endothelial lining. Birch and Brånemark (1969) Scand. J. Plast. Surg. 3:1.

tions against glass in the ear chamber, the authors also observed a shunting to-and-fro movement of blood in some graft vessels. Between 24 and 28 hours after transplantation, slow irregular blood circulation appeared in the original graft vessels. During the subsequent 24 hours most of the grafts had resumed normal circulation (Fig. 20b). Vascular proliferation was observed to commence soon after the development of circulation and to originate from the preexisting graft vessels (Fig. 20c); it reached a peak 6–10 days after grafting. The investigators concluded that the blood flow noted in the graft depends on the vascular connection between the graft and recipient bed and on the host circulation.

In a subsequent study, Birch, Brånemark, and Lundskog (1969) repeated the procedure of transplanting rabbit scrotal skin autografts to the auricular host bed for microangiographic study and reached similar conclusions. Microangiograms showed that the initial graft circulation appears to result from connections between vessels in the recipient bed and large dilated graft vessels. Between 48 and 72 hours following transplantation, capillaries in the host bed penetrate the lower layers of the graft; the small invading vessels are more numerous and penetrate deeper into the donor dermis at the extreme periphery of the graft. However, the capillary invasion does not account for the increased number of all vessels seen in the superficial layers of the graft. Presumably, the new vessels observed in these layers originate from the preexisting graft vessels.

Infrared thermography supplemented by macrophotography (Fig. 21) was used by Birch, Brånemark, and Nilsson (1969) to study the heat emission patterns of vessels of the scrotal skin autograft and its auricular recipient bed. The findings indicate normal heat emission from the host bed vessels under the graft immediately after transplantation. According to the authors, the dilated proliferating vessels in the recipient site slightly increase the temperature of the graft area within the first few days after surgery, provided that the heat emission is not masked by the graft edema.

Another method for assessing the vascular condition and circulation in skin grafts was devised by Marckmann (1966). With a live rat positioned under a microscope and with a television screen amplifier for projection onto a monitor, it is possible to observe the circulating blood in skin autografts and to obtain cinematographic and photographic records. Slow flow could be seen in some areas of the graft 2 days after grafting; the flow velocity becomes normal by the seventh day. The author concluded that the restoration of the microcirculation is attained by connections of the graft blood vessels with those in the recipient bed.

Source of Blood Supply

Many investigative attempts have been made to define the actual source of new blood supply in orthotopic skin grafts by the administration of various dyes, colloidal suspensions, or radioactive substances into the animal vascular system. The conclusions of some authors, including Jungengel (1891), Enderlen (1897), Henle (1899), Davis and Traut (1925), Mir y Mir (1951), and Ham (1962), have already been briefly described.

After intravenous injections of the radioactive isotope ^{32}P into rabbits, Ohmori and Kurata (1960) noted the onset of blood circulation in full-thickness autografts and allografts on the 4th day after grafting. The velocity of the hemic flow is normal in autografts by the 20th day, whereas in allografts the flow diminishes by the 6th day and ceases on the 9th day. Later, Pihl and Weiber (1963) measured the impulse frequencies over the auricular full-thickness skin grafts in rabbits (Fig. 22) after the intravenous administration of ^{32}P partly in the form of a crystalloid and partly in the form of radiolabeled red corpuscles. The data indicate a progressive increase in the vascularization of auto- and allografts until maximum activity is attained

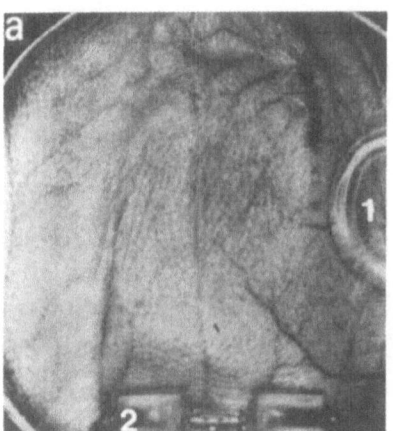
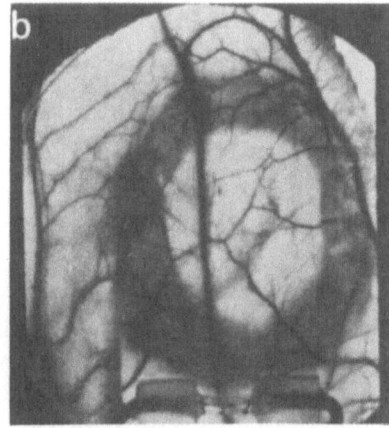
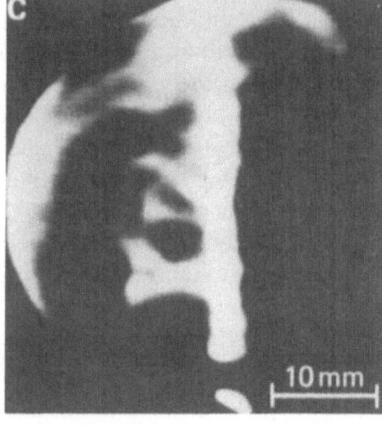

Fig. 21 a–c. Method of studying heat emission patterns of skin vessels in rabbit ear by infrared thermography supplemented by macrophotography. **a.** Macrophotograph with incident illumination. *1* and *2:* probe for temperature calibration. **b.** Macrophotograph with transillumination. **c.** Infrared thermogram of same tissue area. Birch, Brånemark, and Nilsson (1969) Scand. J. Plast. Reconstr. Surg. 3:18.

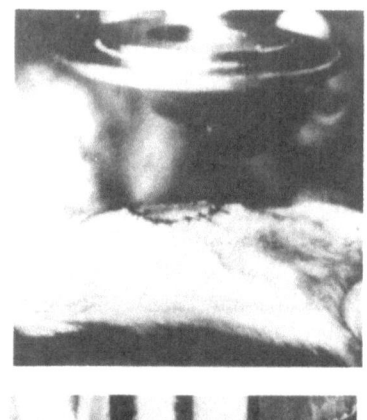

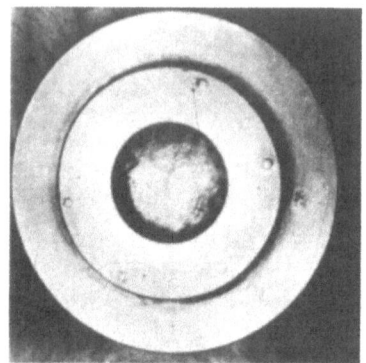

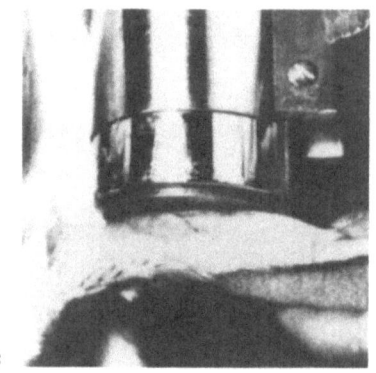

Fig. 22. Application of flanged disc and Geiger-Müller counter over graft for measurement of impulse frequencies after intravenous administration of ^{32}P. Pihl and Weiber (1963) Acta Chir. Scand. 125:19.

by the 5th day. Subsequently, this activity gradually subsides in the autografts, persisting above the level noted in normal skin at 11 days, whereas in the allografts the values diminish when degeneration and the rejection reaction occur. Ohmori and Kurata (1960) and Pihl and Weiber (1963) did not describe the actual process of vascularization.

In vivo microangiographic techniques were employed by Bellman and Velander (1957) and Bellman, Velander, Frank, and Lambert (1964) to define the vascular events in the full-thickness skin graft removed from the auricle of the rabbit and then replaced on its bed. In one experiment (1957) all grafts were rotated 90° before being replaced, and in another experiment (1964) the grafts were not rotated but replaced with exact adaptation. After analyzing the results obtained from both experiments, the authors were unable to state definitely whether the original blood vessels of the transplanted skin participated in the establishment of the definitive vasculature of the graft; however, they wrote that "incorporation of graft vessels into the ambient vessel network is a function of the local hemodynamic status" (Bellman *et al.* 1964).

Šmahel (1962, 1967) used intracardiac injections of a mixture of gelatin and India ink to study the vascular events during the revascularization of

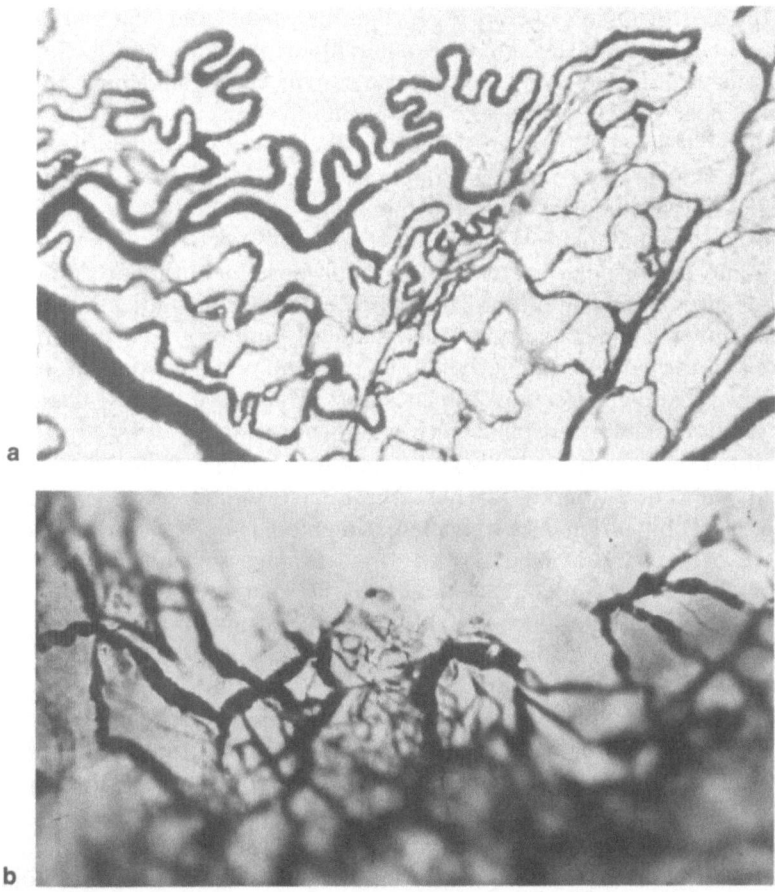

Fig. 23 a and b.   Study of revascularization of skin grafts in rats by means of intracardiac injection of gelatin and India ink. **a.** Total preparation of area in wound bed, second day after transplantation. Detail of architecture of the arcadelike network is seen. **b.** Total preparation of part of the transplant and bed seen from below, third day after transplantation. Fine vessels in the middle of picture are capillary sprouts from arcades; the rest of the more or less filled vessels lying in the focal plane belong to the transplant. Details of the link-ups can be observed. Šmahel (1962) Acta Chir. Plast. 4:102.

skin grafts in rats. He reported that during the first 2 days after transplantation the host capillaries form a rich arcadelike network in the host bed (Fig. 23a). On the following day endothelial sprouts originate from this dense network and invade the graft through the union line (Fig. 23b); on the subsequent days, the host vessels link with the original vascular system of the graft. It has been implied by Šmahel (1962) that if the sprouting of the arcadelike network in the host bed does not develop, the definitive vasculature of the graft will not develop. According to Šmahel and Ganzoni (1970), the revascularization of the skin graft is largely dependent upon the original graft vasculature. However, they were also convinced that under certain conditions the host vessels furnish the major definitive vasculature of the graft. Šmahel and Clodius (1971) have stated that the degree of vascularization of the human skin graft is primarily dependent upon the vascularity of the donor site and secondarily upon the thickness of the graft.

Smith, Ringland, and Wilson (1964) injected silicone rubber at high pressure into the vascular system of the rabbit hosts of auricular skin grafts 1–30 days after transplantation. Their histologic sections indicated, as had those of Converse and Ballantyne (1962), an early and profound sprouting of capillaries in the host bed underlying the graft, numerous capillary sprouts growing in a parallel direction into the graft at about 48 hours, and rapid vascularization of the transplant between 48 hours and 8 days.

In order to include a Y-shaped segment of large well-differentiated artery in the skin autograft for her investigative studies, Stevens (1975) selected the rabbit auricle as a transplantation model. Full-thickness discs of skin were excised by incising down to the cartilage surface on the dorsal aspect and near the tip of the ear where the central artery divides into branches that continue into medial and lateral marginal arteries. Immediately after excision, some of the grafts were returned to the donor sites with their original anatomic orientation (Fig. 24a and b), whereas others were rotated either 90° or 180° before being positioned (Fig. 24e and f).

Preoperative photographs of the vascular system in the area of intended skin grafting under a transilluminated light were compared with the postoperative angiographs of the graft vasculature (compare Fig. 24a with b–d and Fig. 24e with f–h). The vascular pattern of the grafted ear was also demonstrated either by staining the blood vessels with circulating colloidal carbon injected intravenously into the rabbit foreleg or by filling the vessels with India ink by postmortem injections into the ear's central artery.

The experimental data suggest that circulation in the graft vessels is restored on the first or second day after transplantation and continues to improve subsequently. In addition, the large arterial segments within the grafts survive and become permanently joined at the graft periphery to the severed arteries of the adjacent host tissue by well-defined and thin tortuous vascular segments termed "junction vessels." These junction vessels are demonstrable by the angiographic technique as early as 2 weeks; during the following weeks they continue to increase in number. Eventually the arterial segments in the graft become reincorporated into the vasculature of the rabbit auricle. It was also reported that the restoration of circulation, the survival of the graft arterial segments, and the final vascular pattern of autografts are not appreciably affected by the rotation of skin discs at the time of transplantation. The author attributed the successful survival of large arteries in the grafts to the relative rigidity (patency) of the arterial wall, the early reestablishment of circulation, and the favorable hemodynamic position of the grafts in the vascular host bed.

Inosculation of Vessels of the Skin Graft and Host Bed: A Fortuitous Encounter

In 1975 Converse, Šmahel, Ballantyne, and Harper evaluated the vascular patterns of suprapannicular skin autografts in the rat by means of combined procedures of direct skin stereomicroscopy, experimental separation of a graft from its bed (Fig. 25), and supravital intracardiac injection of a contrast medium (Fig. 26). According to the authors, the earliest stereomicroscopic evidence of an initial blood circulation as represented by oscillatory or sluggish movements in the graft vessels at 48 hours is in accord with the concurrent observations of the filling of the graft vessels with India ink (Fig. 26a). Consequently, a delay of 48 hours must elapse for the proliferative host vessels to penetrate the fibrin layer and develop functioning links with the graft vasculature. With an increase in the number and size of functioning anastomoses, accompanied by the gradual dissolution of thrombi, the grafts are completely revascularized between the fourth and fifth days after transplantation; these findings are correlated with complete filling of the graft vascular system with India ink (Fig. 26b) and the stereomicroscopic appearance of brisk blood flow through the graft vessels.

Because only a few vascular anastomoses are found 5 and 6 days after grafting, it was suggested that although numerous capillary sprouts of the host bed contact the graft vessels, only a few of them succeed in forming a functioning anastomosis (Fig. 26b). Furthermore, the presence of a few anastomoses, as demonstrated by the injection procedure, coincides with the stereomicroscopic demonstration of a proportionally denser network of endothelial channels in the graft than in the adjacent host tissue. Moreover, the occasional inosculation revascularizes by means of the anastomotic network of vessels. This has been interpreted as strong circumstantial evidence that graft revascularization is achieved by a dual process of direct connection between the graft and host vasculatures and vascular ingrowth from the host site into the graft.

Split-Thickness Grafts

It has been generally assumed that thin grafts of skin are revascularized more rapidly than thick grafts. The histologic appearance of thin and thick grafts shows that degenerative changes in the transplant depend on the rate of vascularization; the degenerative changes in the transplant appear to be inversely proportional to the rapidity of vascularization. The changes are less apparent in split-thickness grafts, because the invading blood vessels have a shorter distance to traverse through the entire thickness of the donor dermis.

A study employing combined methods of vital skin microscopy and enzyme histochemistry with neotetrazolium chloride and DPNH as reagents was conducted by Converse, Filler, and Ballantyne (1965) in rats. They attempted to define the actual source and development of blood supply in split-thickness skin grafts that were removed, rotated 180°, and immediately replaced on the dermal bed. Before commencing the experiment, the authors had presumed that the revascularization of a split-thickness skin graft transplanted to a suprapannicular bed would be more rapid than that of a full-

---

Fig. 24 a–h. Angiographic study of revascularization of full-thickness graft in rabbit ear. **a.** Preoperative photograph of ear showing the Y-shaped segment of artery *(circle)* included in the graft. ×1.5.

b. Angiogram of the same ear 1 week after graft was replaced in original orientation. The main segment of artery in the graft is partly filled with radiopaque medium. The diffuse radiopacity is due to dilated small vessels in the bed of the graft. ×2.

c. Angiogram of the same ear 3 weeks after grafting. Most of the segment of artery in the graft is now filled by radiopaque medium. The divided end of the central artery in the host tissue tapers to a point *(arrow),* from which arises a thin tortuous channel joining the host and graft vessels. ×2.

d. Angiogram of same ear 11 months after grafting. The segment of the same artery in the graft is now clearly outlined, the diffuse radiopacity has diminished, and junction vessels between host and graft vessels are evident at the lower and the left-hand edges of the graft *(arrows).* ×2. *Inset:* Detail of the left-hand junction vessels showing tortuous channels joining the cut ends of the divided artery. ×4.

e. Preoperative photograph of a second area of grafting *(circle).* The excised disc of skin was replaced after rotation through 90° counterclockwise. ×1.5.

f. Angiogram of second graft 11 months after grafting shows almost complete survival of the segment of artery in the graft. Junction vessels between host and graft are well developed at the lower and the right-hand edges of the graft *(arrows).* ×1.5. *Inset:* Detail of the tortuous junction vessels near the lower edge of the graft. ×4.

g. Preoperative photograph of a third area of grafting *(circle),* which included the Y-shaped division of the central artery and was replaced after rotation through 180°. ×2.

h. Angiogram of third graft 4 months after grafting. Most of the segment of artery in the graft has survived and a junction vessel *(arrow)* is present at the lower edge of the graft. Near the upper edge, the arterial segment *(a)* lies close to but does not join a vein *(v)* at the right-hand side of the graft. ×2. Stevens (1975) Pathology 7:79.

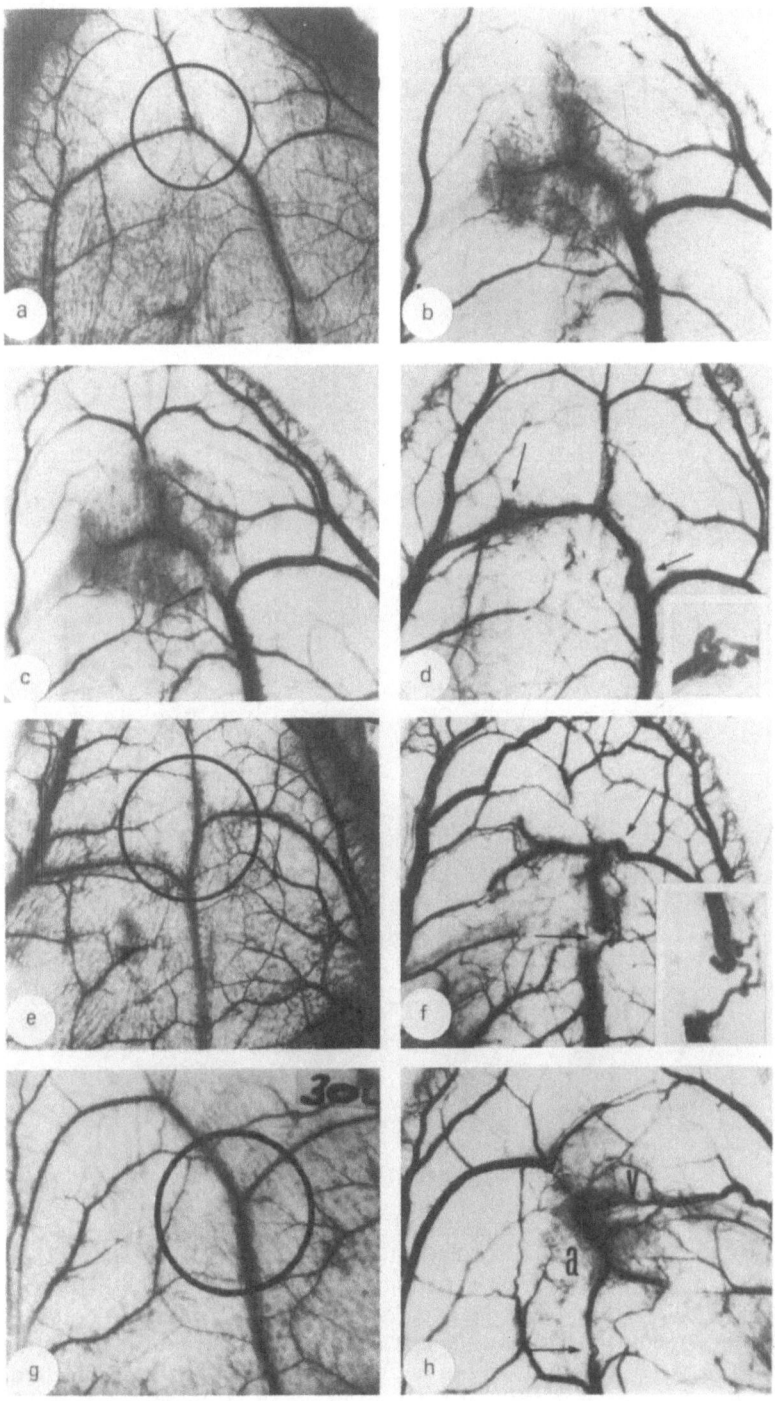

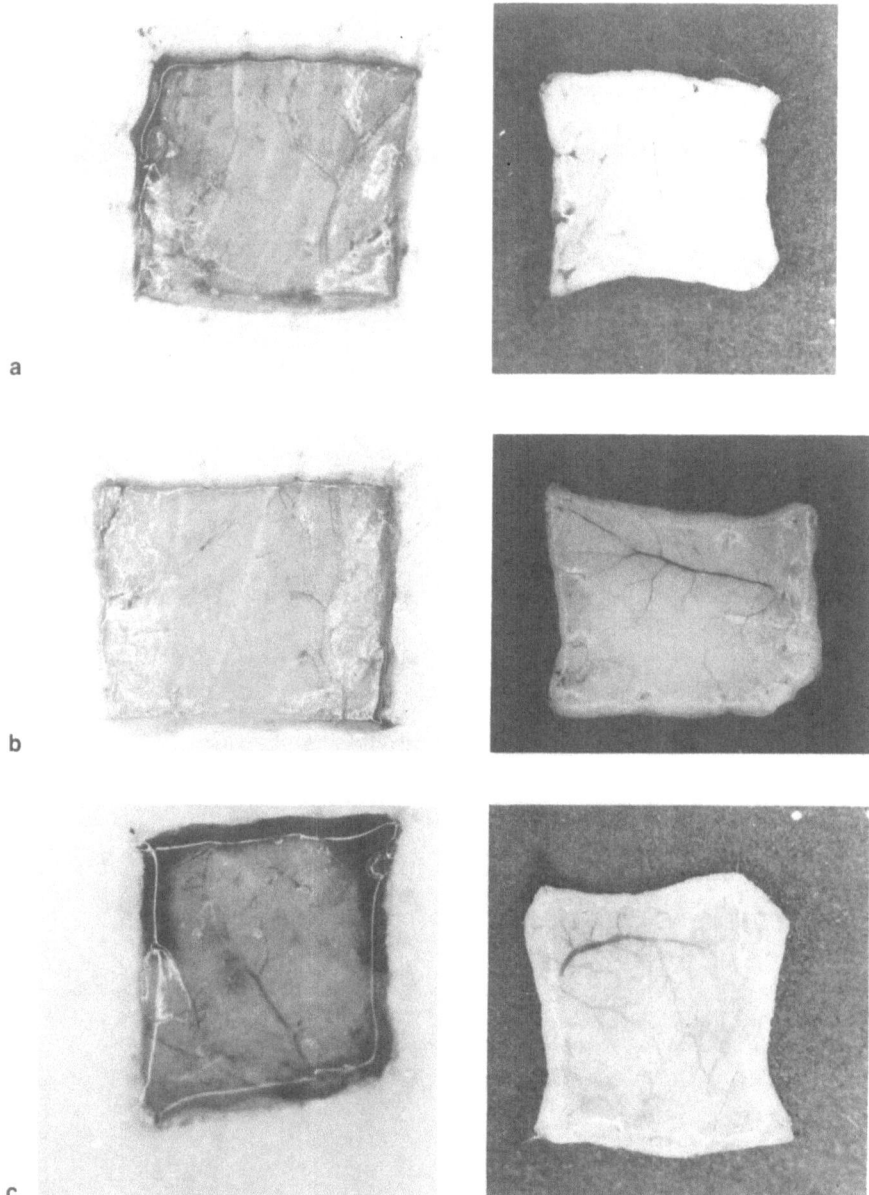

Fig. 25 a–c. **a.** Study of revascularization of suprapannicular skin autograft in rat by means of experimental separation of the graft from its bed. Upturned dermis *(right)* and surface of the bed *(left)* after 1 hour. **b.** After 6 hours. Partial distention of some graft vessels is evident. The bed shows no significant changes. **c.** After 24 hours. There is an increased number, ramification, and distention of the graft vessels and a pool of blood at the margins of the bed. Converse, Smahel, Ballantyne, and Harper (1975) Br. J. Plast. Surg. 28:274.

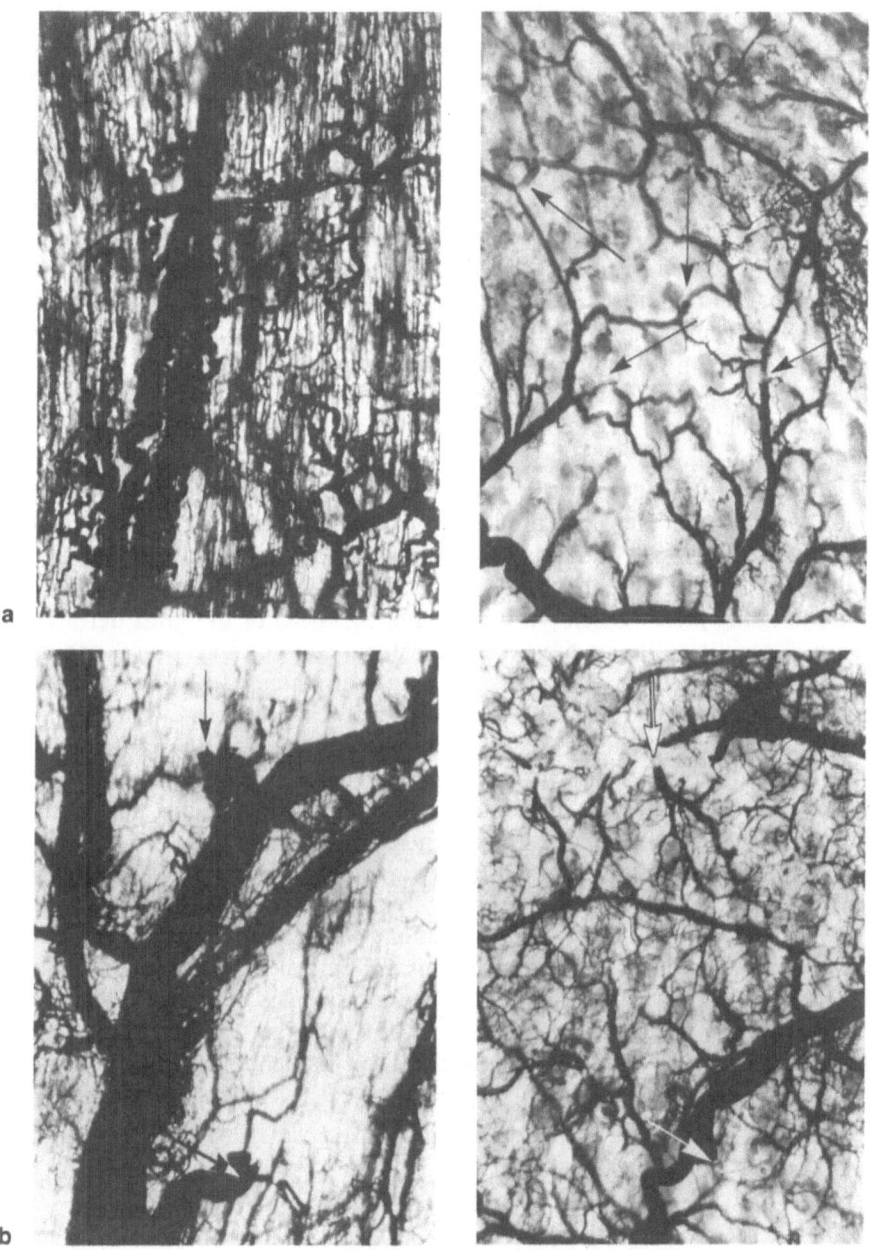

Fig. 26 a and b. Study of revascularization of suprapannicular skin autograft in rat by means of supravital intracardiac injection of a contrast medium. **a.** Opposing areas of the bed *(left)* and the graft *(right)* after 48 hours. Some vessels of the graft are partially or completely blocked by thrombi *(arrows).* ×18. **b.** After 6 days. Well-defined anastomotic units are apparent *(arrows).* ×24. Converse, Smahel, Ballantyne, and Harper (1975) Br. J. Plast. Surg. 28:274.

thickness graft for two reasons: (1) the split-thickness graft is thinner, and the invading vessels from the host have a shorter distance to travel; and (2) the suprapannicular host site contains a rich supply of vessels. Their histochemical data, however, indicated that the new host capillaries originate as endothelial buds (Fig. 27a) from deep-lying distended blood vessels in the upper epymysium of the panniculus carnosus rather than from the host vessels in close proximity to the graft undersurface. The vascular pattern in the host bed is seen to have changed: in comparison to the vasculature noted in the surrounding host tissue, the vessels are very numerous and exhibit greater ramification and dilation. The new vessels show parallel ingrowth from the upper epymysium overlying the pannicular layer to the host–graft junction (Fig. 27b). The complete revascularization with active circulation of the split-thickness graft occurs at the same rate as in the full-thickness graft on a suprapannicular bed.

In contrast to an early and rapid decrease of enzymatic activity in the vessels of full-thickness grafts placed on a suprapannicular bed (Converse and Ballantyne 1962), the delayed and slower loss of activity in vessels in split-thickness grafts implies that the onset and rate of degenerative changes in the original graft vessels vary with the thickness of the graft dermis. In thin grafts, nutrient fluids have a shorter distance to diffuse, and the thinner graft has fewer cellular elements requiring nourishment. As emphasized by Mir y Mir (1951), the rapidity of vascularization and the state of nutrition of the skin graft are controlled by the dermal thickness of the graft and the state of the host site. Woodruff (1960) supported the hypothesis of Mir y Mir that in thin grafts serum imbibition is adequate to maintain the viability of the grafted tissue for several days, and early vascularization is not essential; in thicker grafts, however, early or rapid vascularization is essential for survival.

As mentioned in a previous section, Wolff and Schellander (1965, 1966a), in somewhat similar enzyme histochemical studies, noted that the definitive vasculature of split-thickness grafts in pigs is formed entirely by the ingrowing capillaries from the host (Fig. 17) and the original vessels degenerate. These investigators confirmed the histochemical studies of Converse and Ballantyne (1962), who employed full-thickness skin supra-

---

Fig. 27 a and b *(Opposite).* Vital microscopic study of revascularization of split-thickness graft transplanted to suprapannicular bed. (Sections were incubated with reduced diphosphopyridine nucleotide [DPNH] and neotetrazolium chloride [NT] for 2 hours.) **a.** After 1 day. Note the new endothelial channel originating from host vessel in close proximity to the host panniculus carnosus. ×260. **b.** After 3 days. Note the host vascular ingrowth through the union line into the graft. Union line passes diagonally down from left to right. ×125. Converse, Filler, and Ballantyne (1965) Transplantation, 3:22, © (1965) The Williams & Wilkins Co., Baltimore.

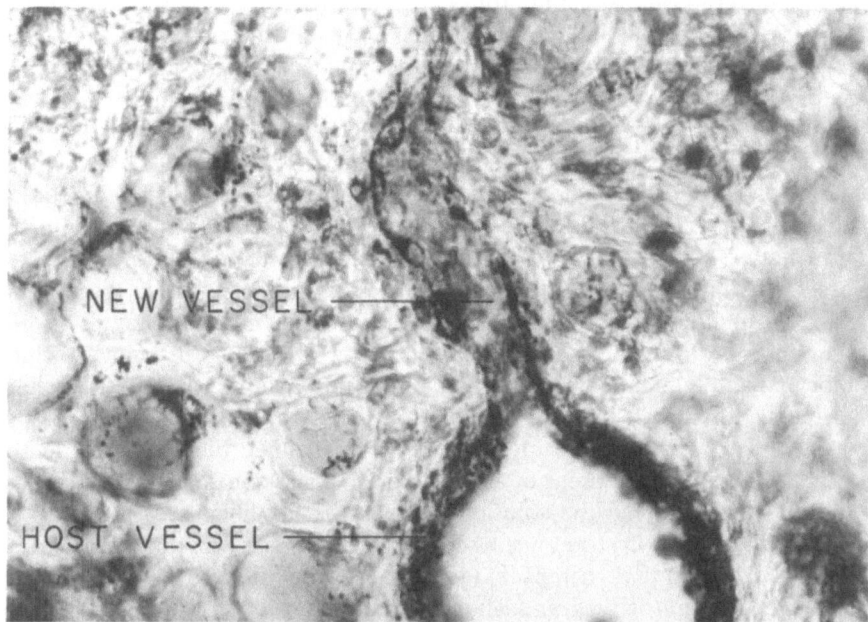

a

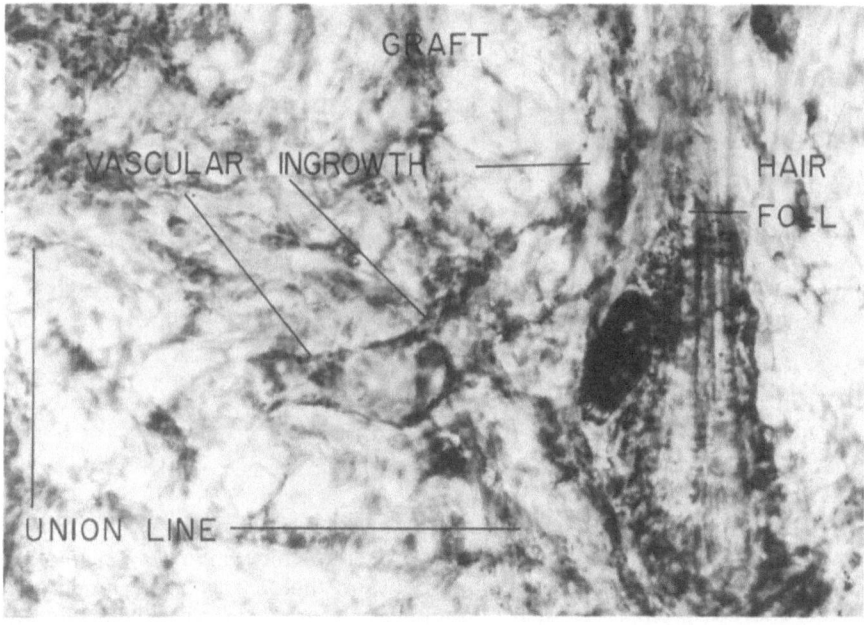

b

pannicular grafts in rats (Fig. 16). Their findings also agreed with those of Converse *et al.* (1965) on split-thickness grafts in rats.

In 1964 Clemmesen introduced an India ink suspension into the vascular system of pigs under forced intracardiac pressure and deduced from the histologic examination that the revascularization of thin split-thickness skin autografts depends largely on the sinuslike channels (Fig. 28) between the vessels of the underlying host tissue and the graft vessels. He concluded that subsequently the sinuslike communications formed by the interstice in the fibrin network at the host–graft junction are transformed into thin-walled vessels, permitting the reestablishment of active hemal flow in the original graft vasculature. Various studies (stereomicroscopy, histology, or histochemistry) of the behavior and fate of skin transplants in animals, chick embryos, and man failed to confirm Clemmesen's findings of sinuslike channels at the host–graft junction. Presumably, excessive intracardiac pressure of the India ink injectant ruptured the newly formed blood vessels at the surface of the recipient areas or at the junction line between the graft and host bed, and thus allowed the solution to form the ink-filled areas.

Using direct skin stereomicroscopy as described by Taylor and Lehrfeld (1953), Woodruff and Simpson (1955) observed numerous capillaries in split-thickness autografts and allografts of rats 4 days after grafting and

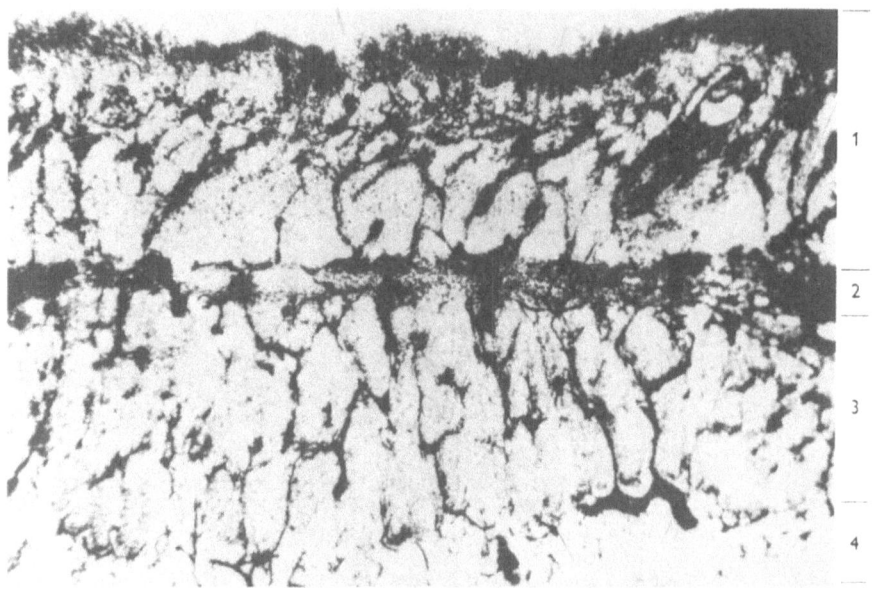

Fig. 28. Split-skin graft with underlying tissue 4 days after transplantation. There are numerous communications between the vessels of the underlying tissue and the graft. *1*, graft; *2*, granulation tissue; *3*, fascia; *4*, muscle. The vessels of the graft are filled with India ink. ×18. Clemmensen (1964) Acta Chir. Scand. 127:1.

increased vascularity in these grafts by 8 days, with more vessels than in normal skin. However, they were unable to discern the condition of the blood flow.

Summary

The present interpretation of the experimental findings is that the early filling of the graft's endothelial spaces with serumlike fluid (previously thought to be plasmalike fluid) is accompanied by the infiltration of erythrocytes, as a result of the anastomosis of graft vessels with host vessels, coupled with the early ingrowth and penetration of host endothelium. These events account for the pinkish tint that appears in human skin within the first 12 hours after transplantation. The color changes gradually to a cherry-red hue in vascularized grafts with well-established blood circulation. The cyanotic color of more slowly revascularized grafts, which reflects poorly oxygenized hemoglobin, is due to incomplete or inadequate hemic flow caused by an embarrassed venous return or drainage from the graft. With time and improved circulation, the color progresses to a cherry-red hue.

Chapter 2

Acute Rejection of First-Set Allografts

It might be expected that a transplant of skin that becomes established and assured of adequate blood supply in a new recipient site is likely to survive intact and to resume its normal function. This expectation is only fulfilled under appropriate conditions.

A skin autograft replaced in its original host bed or transplanted to a new site in the same individual usually continues to survive and to form an integral part of the integument until its survival is terminated by the death of the recipient or by adverse factors such as burns or mechanical damage. Two individuals of ordinary genetic diversity, on the other hand, are unable to receive tissue from each other without its ultimate destruction, a phenomenon referred to as the allograft rejection reaction. After the removal of a skin graft from one individual and its application to another individual, the allograft is initially accepted as though it were an autograft. Its color and general appearance are that of an autograft. However, after a short interval, termed the *latent period,* usually within 10 days, the transplant is rejected amid a series of events characteristic of the immune reaction of allograft rejection.

Since the work of Bert in 1865 all subsequent clinical and experimental investigations have been confined to details of early fluid nourishment and the mode of vascularization in skin transplants. It was not until 1943 that Gibson and Medawar first drew attention to the interactions among the immunologic rejection reaction, the graft breakdown, and the vascular degeneration in the allografts. These data were obtained from the serial comparative histology of auto- and allografts in a female patient. Although this investigation involved a single human subject with extensive loss of skin due to thermal injury and the skin allografts were obtained from a close relative, her brother, the concept of acquired immunity attracted considerable interest in the immunobiology of transplantation. It paved the way for the classic study of Medawar in 1944 and the numerous subsequent investigations on the properties of grafted tissues and organs, interactions between the graft and its host, various manifestations of graft immunity, and many other aspects of transplantation.

The changes occurring in the vascular pattern and morphology of the allogeneic skin form an integral part of the rejection reaction. In the succeeding sections, the various patterns and intensities of graft breakdown in normal and intact recipients are considered with some references to morphologic alterations and survival time of the tissue.

Since allografts may undergo either an acute or chronic rejection process, a composite of acute and chronic rejection episodes is provided in this and subsequent chapters.

Gross Inspection of Grafts In Situ

Gross observation is the most basic and unsophisticated method of evaluating scientific and medical phenomena. Long before the development of microscopes and chemical analyses, it was possible to follow the progress of a graft simply by looking at its appearance. It remains a useful way to gather immediate, general knowledge of the rejection reaction.

From the standpoint of clinical practice, plastic surgeons and clinicians use visual appraisal and touch-palpation as their diagnostic criteria for assessing the condition of the skin grafts and flaps in their human patients at each change of dressings and thereafter at follow-up visits. Close-up photographs (either black and white or color) of the site of surgery are frequently taken for the office files, discussion at clinic meetings, or publication in biomedical journals. With respect to autogenous skin in reconstructive surgery, especially in the treatment of burns or open wounds with loss of skin inflicted by physical agents, extremely few clinicians indeed would resort to histology since it entails excision of graft biopsies. Gibson and Medawar (1943) and Henry et al. (1962) are among the few who took periodic histologic sections, in addition to clinical observations, of auto- and allografts from human subjects. They contributed important information on the sequence of events occurring in human skin grafts. In order to avoid damaging or disturbing the grafts, some investigators, such as Converse and Rapaport (1956), Ceppellini et al. (1966), and McDonald (1968), incorporated direct skin stereomicroscopy as an additional and reliable diagnostic aid. Skin stereomicroscopy is a useful procedure for determining the behavior and vascular system of grafts in situ; unlike histology or histochemistry, it does not disturb or harm the grafted site.

In contrast, investigators working with laboratory animals are able to use various combinations of different diagnostic assay procedures coupled with the gross criteria for assessing the status of grafts. However, when it is desirable to follow intact test grafts as indicators of transplantation immunity and induction of graft tolerance by means of various immunosuppressive agents, diagnostic aids such as histology and histochemistry are not used.

In the 1950's, clinical and research authorities became more critical in their appraisal of the condition and fate of skin transplants. Thus, after reevaluating the problems associated with the application of different criteria, Dammin and Murray, in 1959, categorized the assay methods into gross and microscopic. Gross criteria are based on palpation and the outward appearance of hair growth, skin color, degree of pigmentation, and extent of the graft contraction; the microscopic criteria entail histology, stereomicroscopy, and the use of the sex-chromatin marker. Palpation is helpful in determining the consistency and texture of a graft. Hair growth characteristic of the donor tissue is considered by Dammin and Murray as an absolute criterion of graft survival. In contrast, the color and pigmentation of skin are not comparatively reliable indicators of survival because there is a known tendency for a successful autograft in a black or white person to change from its original color to a darker or lighter hue in either direction.

The visible onset of acute rejection of allogeneic skin in weakly pigmented animal species and humans is manifested by induration, edematous swelling, and transformation from the original delicate pink color to brick red, which soon turns cyanotic. After a short period of extensive hemorrhagic necrosis, the rejected tissue finally sloughs as a hard, dry, and discolored eschar, leaving a variable amount of dermal pad in the recipient bed. During the ensuing reparative process and wound contraction, the collagen pad is temporarily incorporated into the regenerative host tissue, is slowly absorbed, and terminates as a white, thin, linear, and hairless scar.

However, in contrast to the overt signs of acute rejection, it is difficult to determine accurately the behavior and survival end point of grafts that undergo a slower, mild, chronic rejection reaction by their outward appearance. The gross appearance of a chronically rejected graft is different from that of a graft with overt signs of an acute rejection response. The slight induration and mild edema soon decline, and the grafts capable of prolonged survival persist in an autograftlike condition for many days or weeks, but are surreptitiously replaced by host tissue. For these reasons, Billingham and Medawar (1951), Brent (1958), Dammin and Murray (1959), and several others stressed the need for microscopic criteria as a reliable means of scoring survivals.

Raju, Vessella, Grogan, and Conn (1974) discussed the problems of judging skin graft viability by means of gross visual inspection and the discrepancies in the experimental data with regard to graft survival times. To illustrate this point, they designed experiments with inbred rat strains differing at the Ag-B locus, in which the time differential between the rejection of first- and second-set allografts is very short, sometimes as little as 1 day. By correlating the gross and histologic appearance of the grafts, it was determined that the histologic assessment of graft biopsies is the more reliable method of differentiating accelerated rejection from primary rejection in various strain combinations.

Preliminary Histologic Studies

Medawar (1944) described the first study in healthy animal subjects. The behavior and survival times of skin auto- and allografts in rabbits were carefully recorded from histologic examinations of sections prepared from biopsies of full-thickness skin pinch grafts at intervals of 4 days. At 4 days after transplantation, the vascularization, epidermal migration, generalized hyperplasia, and deposition of new collagen in the allografts, coincident with an outward appearance of a delicate pink flush and edematous swelling, are indistinguishable from those of autografts. One early difference between the two types of grafts at this time is the acute infiltration by round cells of native origin in the allograft.

Subsequently, up to 20 or 24 days after transplantation, the autogenous skin (Fig. 29a) shows a progressive period of retrograde differentiation, accompanied by a gradual subsidence of edema and surface color and a progressive return to the appearance of normal skin. In allografts, in contrast, the extent of the subsequent return to a normal pattern depends largely upon the time of onset, as well as the rate of development of the signs of rejection, which vary in intensity from one host to another (compare Fig. 29b with c). Allografts examined at 8 days are usually found to have become swollen with widespread edema and to have changed from a delicate pink hue to brick red, dark red, dirty yellow, or brown. These gross changes are

---

Fig. 29 a–c. *(Opposite)* Histologic sections demonstrating different graft reactions. **a.** A 24-day autograft showing how the pattern of newly formed follicles conforms with that of the old, long since undermined and thrown off by amoeboid and proliferative activities of the epithelium. ×23.

b. An 8-day high-dosage allograft exhibiting the preliminary phases of a mild reaction of breakdown. The graft roof has thickened and stratified, glandular epithelium has hypertrophied, and the primordia of new hair follicles are budding off from epithelium at the bases of the old. Note the wedge-shaped indentations of the roof. Superimposed upon the autograftlike activity, note the acute vascular proliferation and inflammation in the lower reaches of the dermis. A "primary" population of native leukocytes is beginning to invade the graft, and the grossly enlarged lymphatics just below the graft roof already contain many degenerate cells. The fascial planes of the graft bed are not yet distended with edema fluid. ×53.

c. A violent reaction of breakdown in an 8-day high-dosage allograft taking place simultaneously in the whole graft roof. Note the pools of edema fluid in the crests of the dermal papillae. ×89. Medawar (1944) J. Anat. 78:176, Cambridge University Press.

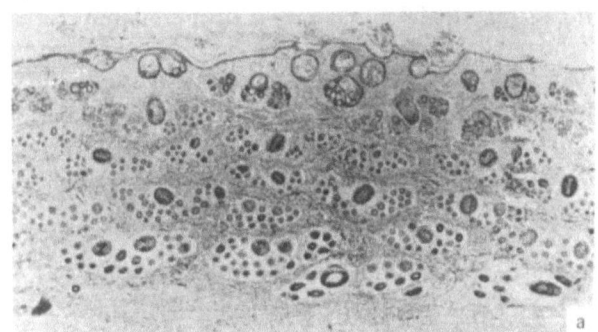

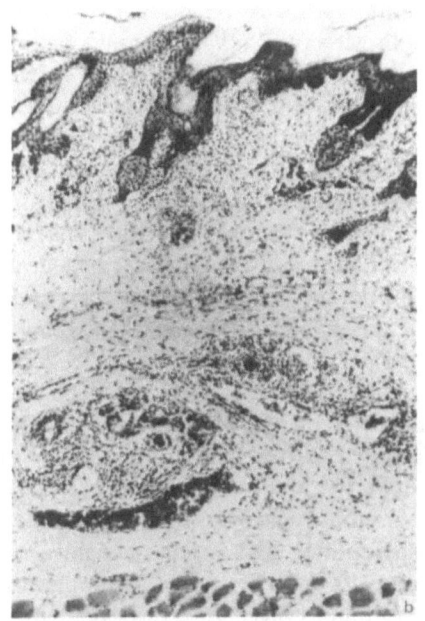

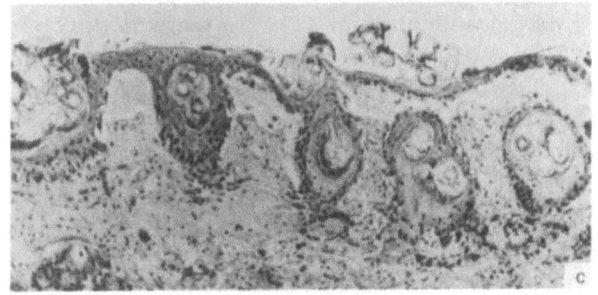

correlated with the histologic picture of a profound but variable cellular infiltration with dilated and engorged blood vessels (Fig. 29b). In a very short time the acute inflammatory reaction attains its peak of violent intensity, coinciding with blood stagnation (Fig. 7b) and complete breakdown of the entire graft vascular and lymphatic systems, followed by necrosis of the graft and shedding of the epidermal cover (Fig. 29c).

According to Medawar (1944), the breakdown of the epidermis and hair follicles in the graft is the principal feature of the rejection episode and is complete within the span of 4 days, from beginning to end. The actual survival time of the graft is estimated by extrapolating the histologic findings, which indicate the limits of epithelial degenerative and necrotic changes seen in a specific graft. The median survival time as calculated by the method of probit analysis for the high-dosage open-style graft exchanged between unrelated rabbits is 10.4 ± 1.1 days.

In later experiments Medawar (1945) studied histopathologic changes occurring in the "fitted pinch" grafts exchanged between unrelated individuals of a heterogeneous rabbit stock. With the exception of a slightly longer median survival time than that observed in the open-style grafts of similar dosage, the sequence of cytologic changes ending in graft destruction closely resembled that described above.

Mention should be made of the fact that the capacity of allogeneic skin to provoke transplantation immunity, as reflected by graft breakdown, does not depend upon the topographic or the structural properties of either the donor or the host tissue. In man and most animals, skin varies considerably in thickness in different parts of the body (Ballantyne and Converse 1966). In the rabbit, the course of events and fate of circular skin transplanted from auricles to the dorsum of normal hosts (Billingham, Krohn, and Medawar 1951) closely resemble those seen in skin grafts removed from the thigh and placed on the thoracic wall (Medawar 1944).

Sparrow (1953) is credited with the first systematic evaluation of skin transplants in male adult guinea pigs selected from a heterogenous stock. Her conclusions were based on gross visual inspection and histologic sections of the auricular skin and body skin grafts placed on the host's chest, beginning on the sixth day after transplantation, and subsequently at 2-day intervals. Grossly and histologically, the course of events observed in the grafts of guinea pigs closely resembles that of grafts in the rabbit described by Medawar (1944), with the exception that the allogeneic inflammatory response is comparatively more subdued in the guinea pig. The explanation by Sparrow (1953) is that the local anaphylactic inflammation (Arthus reaction[1]), so well developed in the rabbit, is not readily seen in guinea pigs.

---

[1] Arthus reaction: A form of heightened sensitivity characterized by the appearance of edematous and subsequent hemorrhagic and necrotic reactions in the site of antigenic administration, produced by interaction of antibodies.

At 6–8 days the autografted tissue is soft and pliable to the touch, shows a pale pink color indicative of a newly acquired vasculature, has the gross appearance of normal skin, and appears flat and depressed below that of the adjacent host skin. In contrast, the allografts are swollen, feel hard, and exhibit a dark, brick-red surface that suggests hemorrhagic necrosis. The biopsies of allografts taken at this time show internal hemorrhage and vascular congestion, together with an acute inflammatory reaction. This is in sharp contrast to the more stable vascular condition and negligible leukocytic infiltration seen in the autografts. Changes in the epithelium, with regard to the progressive epidermal thickening and hyperplasia, are similar in the autografts and allografts up to the rejection time of the latter. Advanced or complete epithelial degeneration, combined with dermal necrosis, is apparent in most of the allografts by the tenth day, the epidermal breakdown preceding the follicular degeneration. As judged by the degree of survival of the graft epithelium following the method of Medawar (1944), the rejection time of the skin exchanges between genetically divergent guinea pigs, as stated by Sparrow (1953), is between 5 and 17 days.

Since the primary purpose of her observations of morphologic changes was to serve as a comparative basis for evaluating the effect of cortisone acetate and ascorbic acid on allograft reaction, no efforts were made by Sparrow to explain the interaction between the pathologic patterns of grafts and the rejection mechanism.

In 1958 Bauer advocated the use of the Padgett-Hood dermatome for preparing split-thickness skin grafts and their host beds in the guinea pig. The experiment was designed specifically to establish evidence of transplantation incompatibility in the guinea pig by means of microscopic comparison of skin auto-, iso-, and allografts applied to two specific inbred strains of animals. The findings show that intrastrain exchanges (isografts) between members of either strain invariably survive, differing in no way from control autografts; this result is grossly represented by a full crop of reversed hair growth, as the donor skin had been rotated when it was grafted.

On the other hand, the interstrain allografts are destroyed rapidly and violently, usually within 7 or 8 days, none surviving beyond 9 days. The earliest indication of a rejection response is increased distention of blood and lymphatic vessels, whose lumina are densely packed with mononuclear lymphoid cells, at 5 days. The events on the following day are reflected by a diffuse mononuclear infiltration into the donor dermis, together with a continued thickening and incipient foamy appearance of the graft's upper epidermal layers. By the seventh day, the original pink hue of the graft has changed to deep red, coupled with patchy breakdown of the epidermal germinative layer. Concurrently, intensified mononuclear invasion and occasional petechial hemorrhages appear in the graft dermis. However, polymorphonuclear infiltration, unlike that in the rabbit, is not a conspicuous feature of the immune response in the guinea pig. Most grafts are rejected at

8 days, as manifested microscopically by the disintegration of the germinative layer of epidermis, frequent subepithelial hemorrhages, and distortion of various dermal structures. Rejection is accompanied by a gross appearance of hemorrhagic, dark brown, and crusted scabs, which slough off within the next 2 days.

Histologic Examinations of Grafted Human Skin

Marshall, Friedman, Goldstein, Henry, and Merrill (1962), by daily clinical and histologic observations, evaluated full-thickness orthotopic auto- and allografts of skin transplanted to normal, healthy, ambulatory human subjects. The preliminary findings served as a control for a subsequent histologic study described in more detail by Henry *et al.* (1962), using similar subjects (see the section on Histologic Studies). Both studies were undertaken because earlier reports on the behavior of human skin grafts were based on biopsies obtained from burned patients (Gibson and Medawar 1943), uremic patients (Dammin, Couch, and Murray 1957), and patients with lymphomas (Green and Corso 1959). Furthermore, most clinicians preferred other diagnostic methods when working with normal humans; for example, Converse and Rapaport (1956) used stereomicroscopy rather than histology in the assessment of the survival time of human allografts.

Marshall *et al.* (1962) stated that, in general, no consistent differences in gross and microscopic appearance are observed between skin auto- and allografts until immediately prior to the onset of immunologic destruction of the graft, although the edema and perivascular infiltration of mononuclear cells seem slightly more pronounced in allografts. The earliest gross evidence of the impending immune response is the reappearance of edema after the reestablishment of a definitive vasculature in the allograft; this is precisely reflected by a histologic picture of invasive perivascular mononuclear cells. According to Marshall and associates, when a graft forms a black eschar 11–14 days after transplantation, the rejection process is completed. With regard to surrounding erythema, the authors stressed that it is not a reliable indication of an allograft reaction because the sutures often elicit a similar inflammatory reaction in autografts. The most striking feature of this work concerns the close correlation between clinical and microscopic findings.

It has been suggested by Marshall and co-workers (1962) that graft edema is the result of the vascular damage caused by the perivascular mononuclear infiltration. This, in turn, implies that the interaction between the vascular permeability and the local delayed hypersensitivity reaction that acts on the vessel wall may play a role in the graft breakdown.

In addition to the findings described in the preceding study, Henry *et al.* (1962) reported that, following complete revascularization of grafted skin in normal humans, the earliest sign of an allogeneic response is the emergence in the graft of a few lymphocytes in the deeper dermal layers around the small venules and the blood vessels supplying the sebaceous glands by the 6th day after transplantation (Fig. 30a). Thereafter, the perivascular infiltration increases in intensity (Fig. 30b) and spreads into the surrounding graft tissue, including the epidermal and pilosebaceous structures. Although the cellular infiltrates are composed mainly of lymphocytes, some histiocytes and eosinophils are noted. During the early stages of the cellular invasion, the blood vessels in the upper dermal layers are distended with blood (Fig. 30c) until the onset of vascular thrombosis in the lower layers of the graft, usually on the 9th or 10th day. Nearly all human allografts undergoing acute changes are completely rejected by the 12th day, as shown by the histologic criteria of necrotic epidermis and early infarction of the graft.

From the histologic lines of evidence that the rejection process is principally vascular and that vascular thrombosis begins before the onset of complete epidermal degeneration in grafts, Henry and associates (1962) concluded that graft destruction can be attributed to the following factors: the specific perivascular lymphocytic invasion acts adversely on the cellular elements of the graft with respect to the vascular endothelium; and a circulating immune agent then induces vascular thrombosis, which leads to hemorrhages, ischemia, and the eventual demise of the graft.

Effect of Cellular Infiltration on the Graft Vessels

Before undertaking an extensive histologic study involving a series of different types of skin grafts in the rat, Waksman, in 1963, formulated a working hypothesis that the timing and the mode of the rejection mechanism may be governed by the density and distribution of the specific graft vascular system (Fig. 31). Various lines of evidence from previous studies laid the basis for this hypothesis. With a few qualifications, the manifestations of autoallergic lesions and other delayed reactions seemed intimately associated with the nature of the vascular network, mainly small veins, at the site of action. To test this hypothesis, orthotopic auto- and allografts of skin removed from the flank and comparable grafts of cervical and auricular skin from the same allogeneic donor were placed in a row on a prepared suprapannicular graft bed on the recipient flank of the rat. Cartilage was included in some auricular grafts.

The results showed that, in contrast to relatively stable conditions and minimal diffuse infiltration of inflammatory cells in control autografts, the first signs of allograft rejection (normally after 5–7 days) occur predominantly in large dilated veins (Fig. 32a), as exemplified by intravascular aggregates and a massive perivascular infiltration of lymphocytes, histiocytes, and other undetermined forms of dark pleomorphic mononuclear cells

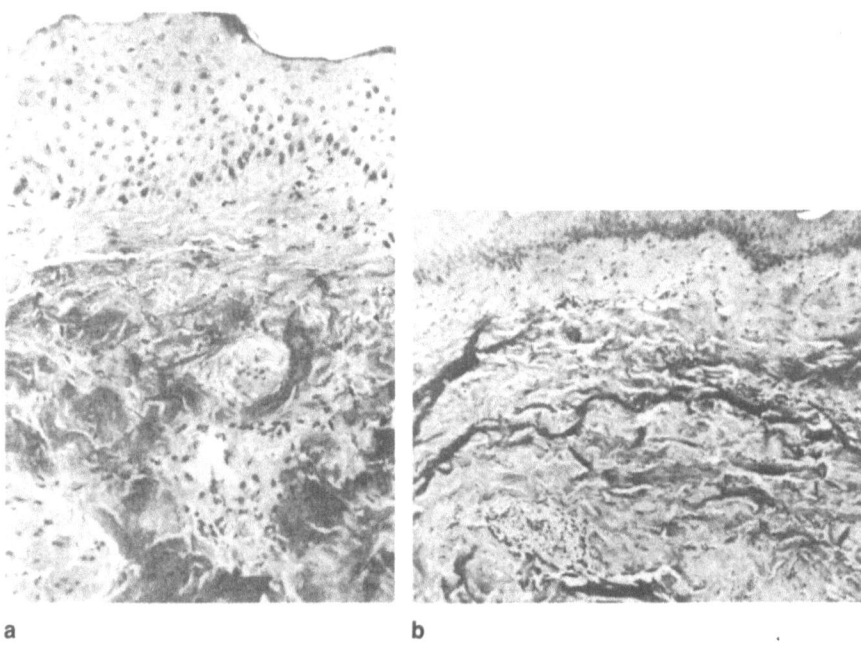

a   b

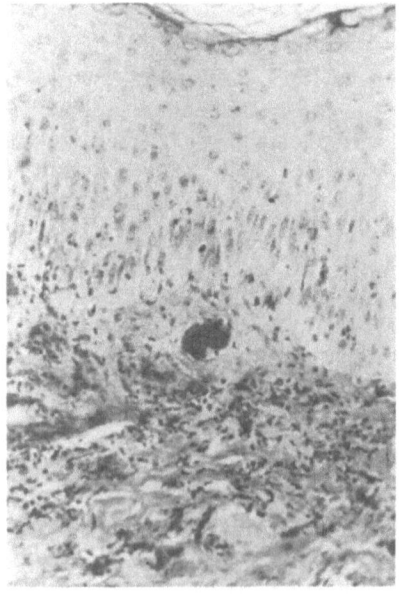

Fig. 30 a–c. Histologic study of allogeneic response in human skin allografts. **a.** The epidermis is intact on the sixth day. The graft has become revascularized but a few small lymphocytes are present around a small venule in the dermis, constituting the first sign of allograft rejection. H & E. ×165. **b.** On day 7 there is a slightly larger collection of lymphocytes around the small venule in the lower dermis. H & E. ×55. **c.** By day 10 vascular thrombosis has occurred in the lower layers of the graft. The blood vessels in the upper dermis are distended with blood. There is ecchymosis and lymphocytic infiltration of the surrounding dermis. The epidermis shows some cellular infiltration but is still intact. H & E. ×165. Henry, Marshall, Friedman, Dammin, and Merrill (1962) J. Clin. Invest. 41:420.

c

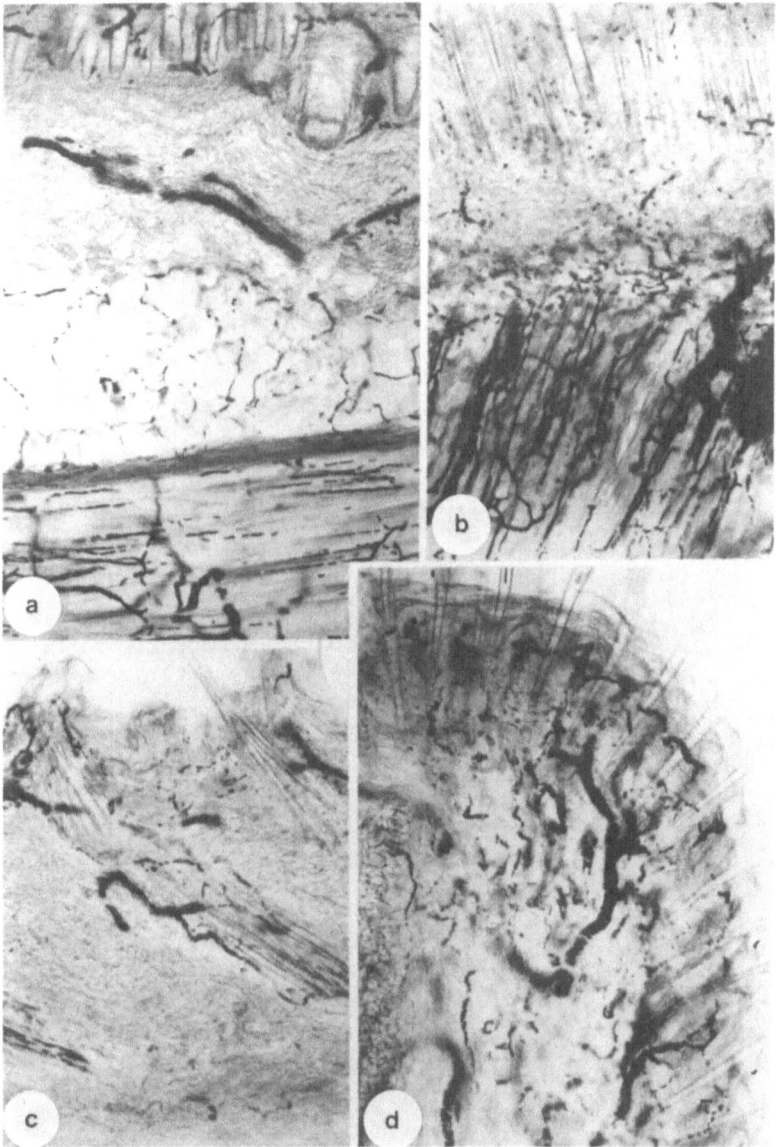

Fig. 31 a–d. Comparison of vascular patterns in several types of skin. Pickworth ben-
zidine stain. ×75. **a.** Guinea pig flank skin, showing large veins in dense dermal connective
tissue and venules in upper zone of dermis between follicles, as well as veins in underlying
panniculus. **b.** Rat flank skin, showing large veins in panniculus and at base of dermis but an
almost total absence of veins in the dermis proper and subepidermal region. **c.** Rabbit flank
skin, showing vascular pattern similar to that of guinea pig, however, with fewer veins in the
dense dermis. **d.** Rat ear, showing venules between follicles and larger veins throughout
deeper connective tissue. Waksman (1963) Lab. Invest. 12:46, © (1963) U.S.–Canadian
Division of the International Academy of Pathology.

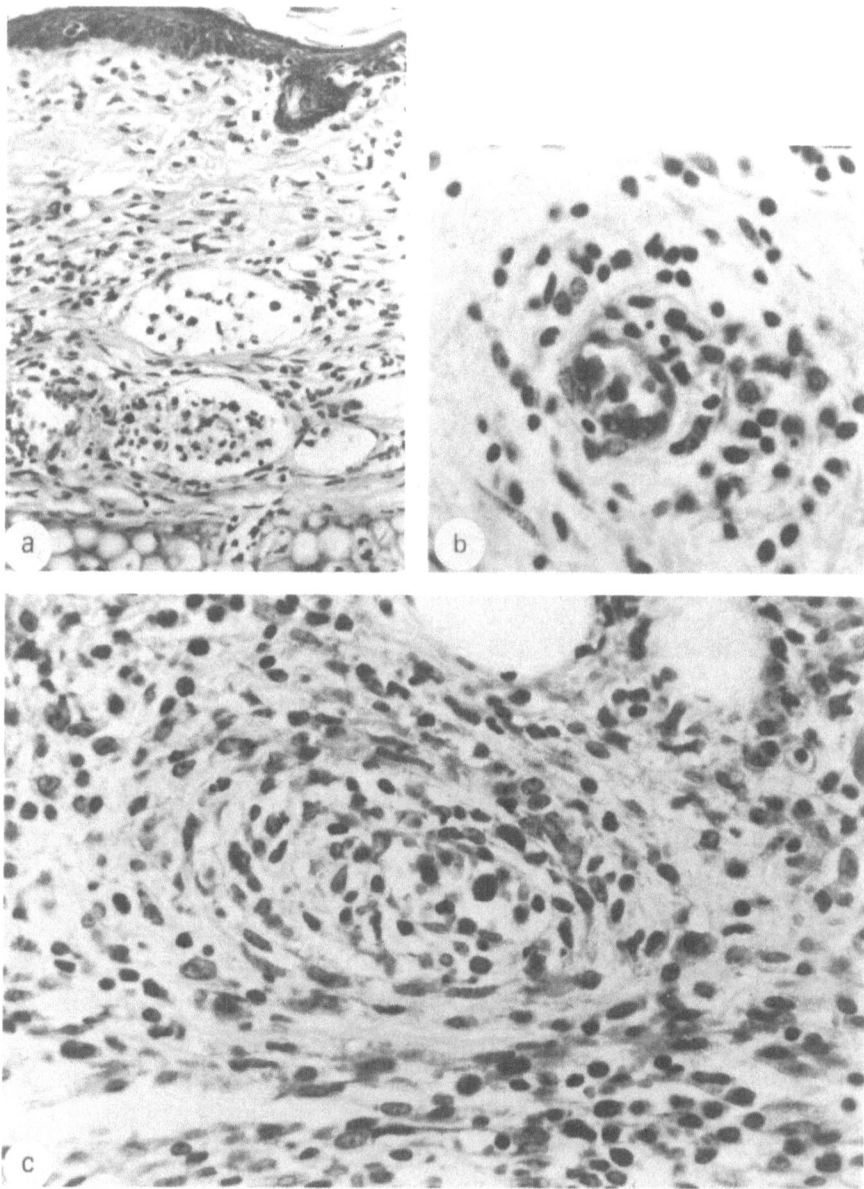

Fig. 32 a–c. Early vascular lesions in skin allografts in rats. **a.** Ear skin graft at 5 days, showing formation of cellular "thrombus" in large veins of graft. Lower vein shows thrombus in central portion and vasodilation and stasis of portion immediately to the left. On serial section, it was found that these are parts of the same vein. ×160. **b.** Flank skin allograft at 7 days, showing characteristic perivenous infiltration of mononuclear cells. Lumen of vein remains patent and endothelium is intact. ×370. **c.** High-power view of artery in flank skin allograft at 7 days. Vessel remains patent although architecture of vessel wall is destroyed. Part of endothelium is intact, but larger part is extensively vacuolated and nuclei have disappeared. ×325. Waksman (1963) Lab. Invest. 12:46, © (1963) U.S.–Canadian Division of the International Academy of Pathology.

(Fig. 32b). The intensity, site, and development of the early cellular response appear to depend largely upon the graft vascularity, particularly the veins, in the skin grafts obtained from different parts of the body.

Such events rapidly lead to progressive obliteration and destruction of the vessels by mononuclear cells (Fig. 32c) at 7–10 days, followed by invasive destruction of the epidermis, pilosebaceous structures, and all existing arterial and venous vessels in the donor skin. The infiltrating cells appear to be responsible for the extensive damage to the endothelial walls of the graft vasculature. The intraluminal obstruction and destruction of the vessels by the invading host cells bring about cessation of the circulatory blood and hemorrhage, resulting in the ischemic death of the graft.

It was suggested by Waksman (1963) that the death of a skin allograft is brought about by the intensive accumulation of host mononuclear cells and direct cytopathogenic action by these cells on the graft blood system, not by the effects of the host antibody on the endothelium. Thus, according to Waksman, the breakdown of the graft epidermis and hair follicles and the cessation of blood flow—selected as the salient criterion of the rejection process by Medawar (1944) and Taylor and Lehrfeld (1953), respectively— are more or less the derivative changes occurring late in the rejection process.

Experimental Vital Skin Microscopy

Taylor and Lehrfeld, in 1953, and more specifically in 1955, called attention to the inherent weakness of the gross observation and histologic analysis of grafts. They introduced the direct stereomicroscopic method (Fig. 10) for observing grafts in situ under incident light on successive days, by which the changes in the blood vessels and the condition of blood flow can be easily seen. By this technique, the authors showed that in the rat there is very little divergence in the vascular pattern between autografts and allografts during the first 4 days after transplantation (see Fig. 12b–e and the discussion in text). However, at the end of this period the vessels in the graft become more numerous and exhibit greater distention than those in the adjacent host skin. Thereafter, the autograft vasculature progressively resumes the vascular pattern of normal skin, while the extent of the subsequent return of the allograft blood system depends largely on when rejection occurs. The sequence of events leading to the allograft breakdown is preceded by multiple punctuate thrombi, a slowing down and eventually a complete cessation of circulating blood within the graft vessels (Fig. 12f), and vascular disruption resulting in the extravasation of blood (Fig. 12g and h), usually 7–9 days after transplantation, with a mean survival time of 8.3 days in the rat. Taylor and Lehrfeld (1953) concluded that, since the onset of vascular disruption occurs before the degeneration and necrosis of grafted tissue, the endothelium of the capillaries is the first site of attack by immunologic agents.

Woodruff and Simpson (1955) introduced a suitable method of preparing split-skin grafts, either as fitted or open-style grafts, with a small dermatome of the Padgett type for application to rats. They also provided data concerning the sequential reactivity of the fitted split-thickness transplants. Grossly and histologically, and by vital skin microscopy of the capillary pattern, the allografts were found to heal and to react like autografts for approximately 12 days (compare Fig. 33a–c with e and f). However, unlike Taylor and Lehrfeld (1953), Woodruff and Simpson could not discern the state of the capillary blood flow even in autografts and could not pinpoint the capillary stasis in the tissue undergoing rejection.

At 4 days after surgery the capillaries appeared more numerous in the grafts compared to normal skin, while the histology of grafts closely resembled normal skin. At 8 days the capillary network had become more extensive in the grafts and the vessels much more numerous but not very different in caliber when compared to the host skin. Numerous dilated blood vessels and a small amount of newly formed connective tissue appeared at the line of demarcation between graft and host. Histologically, the graft epidermis showed some thickening but not on the scale described by Medawar (1944) in open-style grafts in rabbits.

However, unlike autografts, which in due time resumed the gross and histologic characteristics of intact skin, the earliest histologic evidence of an altered response toward foreign skin was a slight but definite round cell infiltration at 8 days. This inflammatory reaction, while never as apparent as that in rabbit grafts as described by Medawar (1944), was intensified at 12 days (Fig. 33f), with a slight thickening of the graft epidermis. At this stage, the allogeneic epidermal and follicular cells stained less readily than those in the autografts but did not show gross degenerative changes.

In contrast to the brick-red appearance of the rabbit allografts, the rat grafts were grossly pale and felt rigid on touch-palpation. According to Woodruff and Simpson (1955), while skin microscopy usually indicated the capillary hemorrhage reported by Taylor and Lehrfeld (1955), it did not invariably occur, and the survival time of a graft is liable to be overestimated if too much reliance is placed on this criterion. Meanwhile, the histologic observations showed complete breakdown of the graft epithelium and early replacement of the graft remnants by the granulation tissue from the host bed (Fig. 33g). The authors estimated the survival time of the grafts to be 13 or 14 days.

In 1957, Castermans studied the behavior of skin grafts in mice through a modification of vital microscopy under incident light illumination (see page 23). Comparative examinations of auto- and allografts showed that the first vascular changes associated with the allograft breakdown begin 8–9 days after transplantation. The changes consist of irregular and enormous dilation of the graft vessels, followed rapidly by thrombosis and perivascular hemorrhages. In contrast, the capillary network in the autografts progressively assumes a normal vascular pattern.

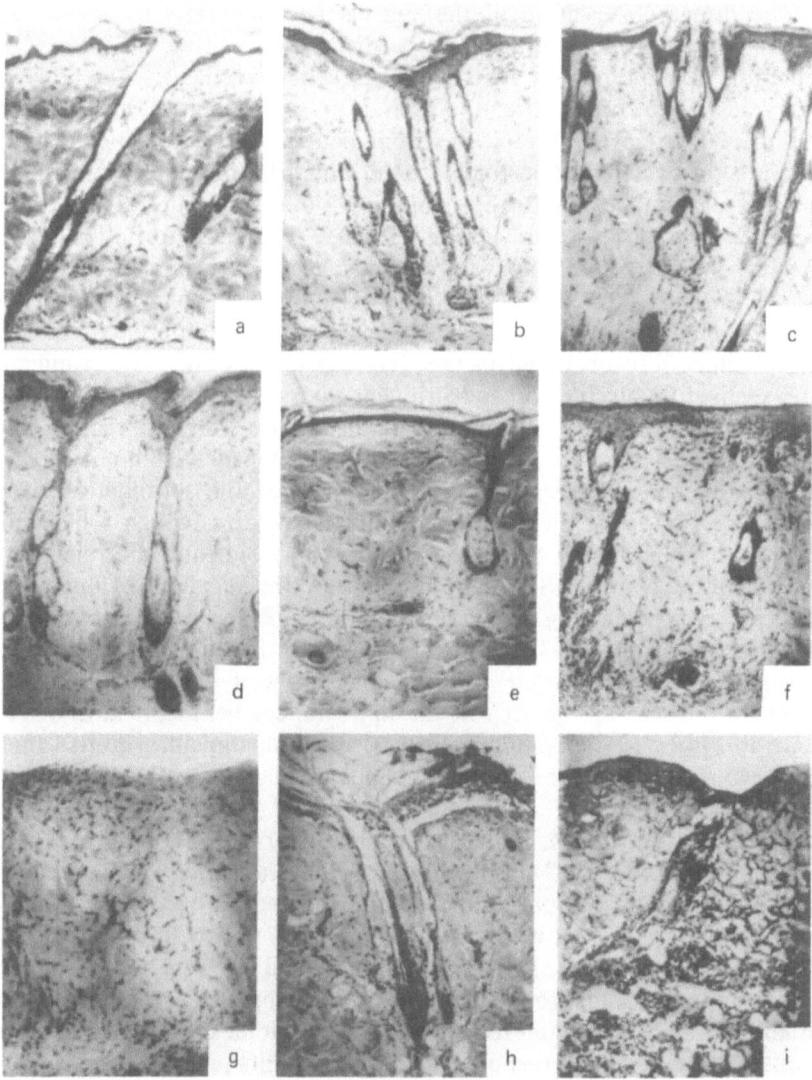

Fig. 33 a–i. Histologic sections of grafts in rats. ×55. **a–d.** Autografts after 4, 8, 12, and 16 days, respectively. **e–g.** First-set allografts after 4, 12, and 16 days, respectively. Round cell infiltration is apparent in the 12-day graft, and the 16-day graft has been completely destroyed and is being invaded by granulation tissue. **h and i.** Second-set allografts after 4 and 7 days, respectively. Breakdown is almost complete in the 4-day graft. Woodruff and Simpson (1955) Plast. Reconstr. Surg. 15:451, © (1955) The Williams & Wilkins Co., Baltimore.

The direct observation of the vessels in skin grafts by means of a dissecting microscope as practiced by Taylor and Lehrfeld (1953) was also adopted by Ballantyne and Converse (1957) for investigating the effects of skin cycles on the vascularization and survival of allografts in the rat. In addition, two types of grafts, suprapannicular and subpannicular, were studied. Skin cycles can be readily determined by periodic cycles of hair growth in such animals on the basis of the various age groups: 22, 32, and 42 days. These age groups were selected because, according to Butcher (1934), at 22 days the hair follicles are at a resting stage, at 32 days the follicles have resumed growth, and at 42 days the hair follicles have attained their maximum depth into the dermis. While appreciable differences in mean survival time were observed in the different age groups, suprapannicular grafts seemed to survive somewhat longer than subpannicular grafts of the corresponding age group. When all the hair follicles were at a resting stage, as in the 22-day-old rats, the survival time of allogeneic skin was longest. The survival time of grafts was shortened after the termination of the quiescent period, as in the 32-day-old animals. When new hair follicles had achieved their maximum depth, as in the 42-day-old rats, the rejection of skin allografts occurred more rapidly than in either of the previously mentioned groups, coinciding with the rejection time previously reported by Taylor and Lehrfeld (1953) in adult rats. Except for the survival time, the gross and stereomicroscopic examinations showed very little difference among these three age groups in the appearance, behavior, and vascular events in either the subpannicular or the suprapannicular grafts. In the 42-day-old rats, brisk blood circulation appeared somewhat later, usually on the fourth day.

In these experiments, Ballantyne and Converse (1957) reported, as did Taylor and Lehrfeld (1953) in the adult rat, that the earliest evidence of the impending rejection episode is the dilation of the graft blood system, followed by a sluggish flow with clumped elements. A few thrombosed areas appear shortly thereafter, particularly in the small capillary loops, and subsequently spread rapidly to the larger vessels. Complete cessation of circulation and vascular disruption follow, usually by the next day. Grossly, after the onset of the rejection response, the graft exhibits progressive changes in color, turning various shades of red, yellow, or green, and feels rigid on touch-palpation. It is sometimes crusted and escharified.

Additional experiments were undertaken by Ballantyne and Converse in 1959 to determine the relationship of hair-skin cycles and the survival times of allografts of rats of three age groups: 3, 6, and 12 months old. Attempts were also made to study any difference in the course of events between sub- and suprapannicular grafts in the corresponding age groups and the influence of hair plucking on the graft rejection time. The results showed that the grafts in unplucked rats of all age groups follow the postoperative course and survival times observed by Taylor and Lehrfeld (1953) and Ballantyne and

Converse (1957) in 42-day-old rats. In the 12-month-old recipients, the caliber of the blood vessels of the subpannicular grafts is slightly larger than that of the suprapannicular grafts. This increased dilation also appears earlier in the subpannicular skin. However, in contrast, the mean survival time is decreased consistently in the corresponding age group of plucked rats. It has also been found that the older the rat, the greater the dilation of vessels in the plucked animalₛ. In the unplucked animals, beginning with the 42-day-old rats as reported by Ballantyne and Converse (1957), there is no decrease in the mean survival time of allografts with increasing age.

Stereomicroscopic Studies of Human Grafts

Based on periodic gross and stereomicroscopic examinations of full-thickness skin grafts (Figs. 13 and 34) in the human (see the section on Stereomicroscopic Studies in Chapter 1), Converse and Rapaport (1956, 1957) discerned the initial divergence in appearance, behavior, and vascularity between the autografts and allografts at 6 days after grafting (Figs. 13c and 34d). The characteristically dilated vessels seen in the autografts during the first few days after transplantation progressively become less numerous and of smaller caliber, returning to a normal vascular pattern; in allografts, the rejection phenomenon is an orderly progression of events beginning with secondary erythema (Fig. 34d) around the affected graft by day 6. This change is closely associated with stereomicroscopic evidence of progressive dilation and diminished blood flow of the graft vessels. By day 8 or 9 the allograft appears cyanotic (Fig. 34e) and the blood circulation has ceased completely (Fig. 13d), followed by thrombosis of the graft capillaries within 24 hours (Fig. 13e). In the next 24 hours, the vessel walls rupture, extravasation of blood occurs (Fig. 13f), and eventual graft necrosis (Fig. 34f) and sloughing follow. This sequence of events leading to the rejection of human skin allografts is heralded by the progressive arrest of blood flow that began 24 hours before.

The rejection time of allografts in man described by Converse and Rapaport (1956), particularly in terms of stagnation of blood circulation in the graft vasculature, followed by vascular breakdown and graft necrosis, is in close agreement with the survival time in lower forms. Indeed, Billingham, Brent, Medawar, and Sparrow (1954) drew attention to the fact that the survival times of skin allografts of comparable dosage in chicks, mice, rats, guinea pigs, rabbits, and cattle are within the range of 7–10 days, regardless of the survival criteria.

In 1966 Ceppellini et al. considered stereomicroscopy to be particularly useful in assessing behavior and survival of human skin exchanges between unrelated individuals, between parent and child, and between siblings. They tested orthotopic full-thickness skin grafts in healthy human volunteers divided into the three matched groups, with particular attention paid to the genetic relationship between donor and recipient, and also to the role of ABO-incompatibility in the rejection mechanism. After successful vascularization of grafts in an unrelated recipient by 6–7 days after transplantation, the capillary loops located in some discrete areas near the graft surface begin to evince minute dilations, usually not earlier than 10 days. These vessel changes, termed the "capillary ectasias," are believed to be the

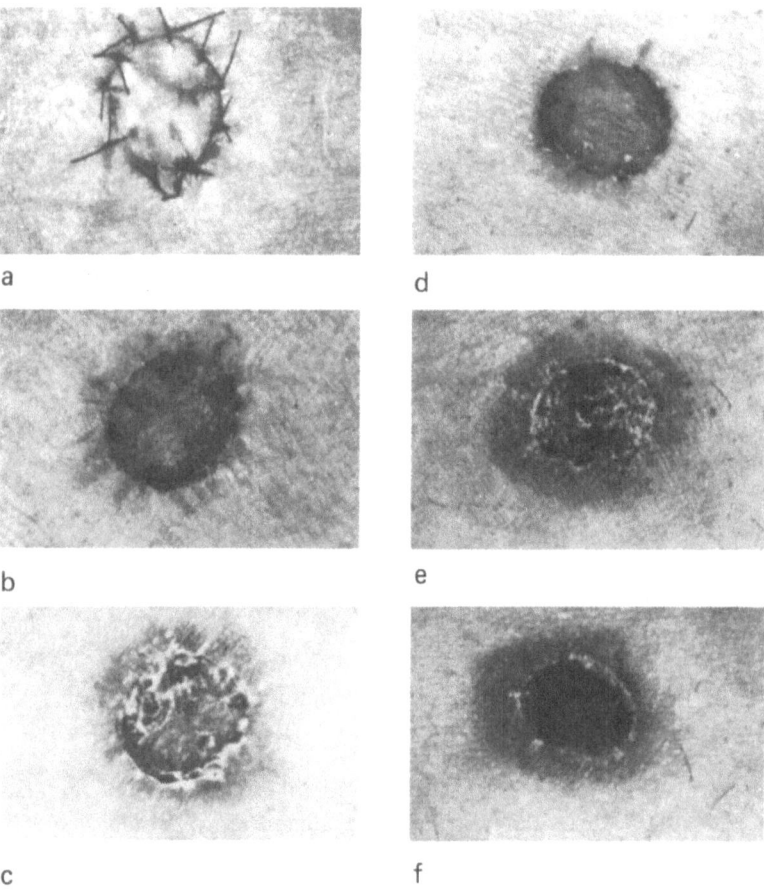

Fig. 34 a–f. Gross appearance of skin autografts and allografts at various stages after transplantation. **a.** Graft 24 hours after transplantation. **b.** Autograft on day 4. **c.** Autograft on day 7. Surface epithelium is being desquamated. Note merging of graft and host epidermis. **d.** Allograft on day 6. Note the secondary erythema appearing around the graft. **e.** Allograft on day 9. The graft has a cyanotic appearance and the secondary erythema has increased. **f.** Allograft on day 12. The graft is becoming escharified. Converse and Rapaport (1956) Ann. Surg. 143:306.

visible manifestations of early vascular damage. During the next 2–4 days, ectasias progressively spread over the graft upper layers, accompanied by petechiae along the capillary network and followed suddenly by the discernible appearance of the distal parts of the capillaries throughout most of the graft tissue. Grossly, the graft color concurrently changes from red to purple and eventually shows signs of hemorrhaging. These changes, as suggested by Ceppellini and associates (1966), who called them "capillary thromboses," are similar to the cessation of intracapillary blood flow described previously by Converse and Rapaport (1956).

Perivascular hemorrhages then follow, becoming grossly apparent within 24 hours. Based on the stereomicroscopic observations of capillary thrombosis selected as a rejection criterion, the mean survival time for 54 unrelated donor grafts was 12.1 days, but was improved in the other two matched groups, whose results are reviewed in Chapter 3. The data also imply a close association between decreased survival time of grafts and ABO-incompatibility, particularly when an A_1 graft is applied to an O recipient, which can cause a white (avascular) graft type of rejection even in the first-set skin grafts.

McDonald (1968) described two distinctly different patterns of rejection, designated as nonhemorrhagic and hemorrhagic, in first-set skin allografts of healthy human subjects. Stereomicroscopically, after successful revascularization, the progressive signs of a graft undergoing the nonhemorrhagic form of rejection are (1) dilations and gradual disorganization of the graft vasculature, beginning 7 days after transplantation, (2) gradual vascular disruption, (3) dry necrosis, and, finally, (4) escharification. In addition, the rejection procedure is regularly accompanied by edema, variable in extent and in the time of appearance. Although there is a complete absence of hemorrhage in grafts exhibiting the pure nonhemorrhagic type of rejection, a small amount of extravasated blood may occasionally be seen along the course of distended vessels in other grafts.

Grafts undergoing a hemorrhagic pattern of rejection survive at least 1 day longer than grafts undergoing nonhemorrhagic rejection. The superficial desquamation of the graft surface has sufficient time to be complete, thus exposing a thin, shiny epidermis. Instead of vascular dilation and a gradual disruption, which are features of the nonhemorrhagic type of rejection, fine delicate blood vessels predominate until the sudden occurrence of a massive hemorrhage, reflecting the graft rejection. McDonald (1968) also reported a combination of nonhemorrhagic and hemorrhagic rejection in another group of first-set allografts, in which the vascular changes of nonhemorrhagic rejection were superseded by hemorrhagic necrosis.

It was concluded that the survival time of skin allografts could not be attributed to host immunity alone in this series of human subjects, but rather that the pattern of rejection response is determined by histocompatibility between donor and recipient in combination with host immunity.

Assessment of Graft Behavior by a Combination of Various Assay Methods

The behavior of autologous and allogeneic transplants of mouse and rat skin was investigated by Rolle, Taylor, and Charipper (1959) using a combination of the following four procedures: (1) daily gross and stereomicroscopic examinations of the grafts in situ as developed by Taylor and Lehrfeld (1953); (2) routine histologic preparations; (3) cardiac injections into the vascular system of host animals with suspensions of India ink after the method of Scothorne and McGregor (1953); and (4) intravenous injections of a diffusible dye, bromophenol blue. The earliest criteria of the rejection process were exemplified by blood engorgement and distention of the graft blood vessels immediately before the slowing down and eventual cessation of hemal flow in the graft; there was no evidence of blood clots. The authors attributed the slowing and eventual cessation of flow to the engorgement of vessels. Blood circulation generally ceased 7–8 days after grafting, rapidly followed by the degeneration of the formed hemic elements and endothelial cells (Fig. 35), progressing downward through the depth of the graft dermis from the dermoepidermal junction.

Because the degenerative changes in the graft epidermis and dermis occurred 24–48 hours after complete hemal stasis, the authors ascribed the graft destruction to the vascular failure, probably generated by an Arthus-type reaction.

On the basis of daily gross and stereomicroscopic examinations, confirmed by histopathology, of full-thickness skin auto- and allografts in guinea pigs, Guthy, Billote, and Burke (1974) concluded that the process of graft destruction is mediated by three mechanisms, of which two are immunologic and one is nonimmunologic: (1) early endothelial rejection, which appears between 6 and 9 days; (2) late epithelial–endothelial rejection between 9 and 10 days; and (3) intercepted vascularization due to a combination of technical failures and immunologic factors.

In the early endothelial type of rejection, after successful revascularization by 4 days after transplantation (reviewed in more detail on page 24), the grafts remain in a viable condition until the onset of the rejection response, between 6 and 9 days, as shown by cyanosis accompanied by an intense polymorphonuclear leukocytic infiltration into graft vessels but not into the graft epidermal cells. These events are rapidly followed within 12–24 hours by edema, induration, and desquamation of the graft surface, coincident with extensive vascular damage. During this time the endothelial cells, whether intact or lysed, are separated from the basement membrane and aggregate within the vessel lumen. In contrast, the epidermal cells continue to appear unaltered upon histologic examination. During the next 24 hours, vascular lesions become more intensified, with histologic evidence of platelet aggregation and extensive occlusive thrombosis. At this time, the

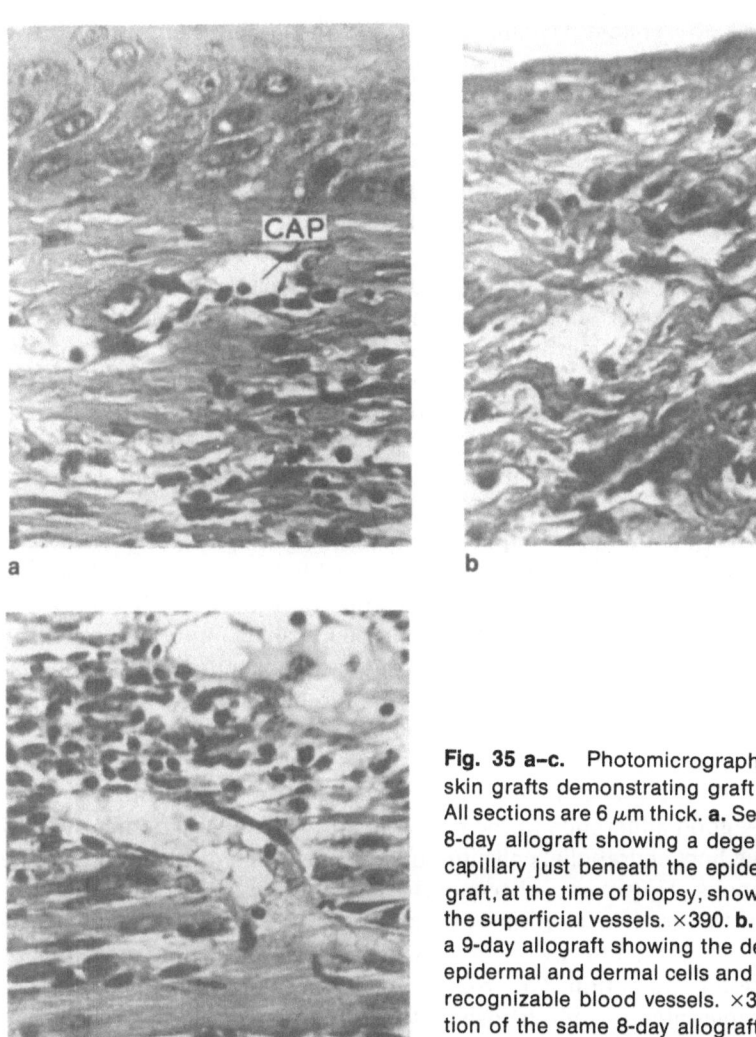

Fig. 35 a–c. Photomicrographs of rodent skin grafts demonstrating graft rejection. All sections are 6 μm thick. **a.** Section of an 8-day allograft showing a degenerated capillary just beneath the epidermis. This graft, at the time of biopsy, showed stasis in the superficial vessels. ×390. **b.** Section of a 9-day allograft showing the degenerated epidermal and dermal cells and the lack of recognizable blood vessels. ×390. **c.** Section of the same 8-day allograft shown in panel a, showing a dermal capillary containing some hemolyzed and some normal erythrocytes and slightly pyknotic leukocytes. ×390. Rolle, Taylor, and Charipper (1959) J. Cell. Comp. Physiol. 53:215.

graft epidermal layer exhibits multiple, coalescent, intraepidermal blisters indicative of ischemic damage due to vascular damage and occlusion. However, unlike allografts, after vascularization control autografts resume the conditions of surrounding host skin.

Because the intensive infiltration of polymorphonuclear leukocytic infiltrates causes extensive damage and intraluminal obstruction of the graft vessels, with consequent ischemic necrosis of the graft epidermis, Guthy *et al.* (1974) suggest that the immune reaction seen in this type of graft rejection is principally vascular, brought about by humoral antibodies acting on the endothelium, not on the epidermal cells, similar to Arthus-type reaction.

In the late epithelial–endothelial type of rejection, the grafts, if effectively revascularized by 4 days, demonstrate persistent hyperemia, occasional cyanosis, and varying degrees of edema during the next few days. By 9–11 days, the grafts become cyanotic, swollen, and indurated, with complete cessation of blood flow in the graft vessels. Histologically, the graft is characterized by small lymphocyte infiltration in the basal and prickle cell layer of the allograft epidermis, epithelial lysis, and complete separation of the edematous graft epidermis from its subjacent dermis. Concurrently, the blood vessels also undergo infiltration of small lymphocytes, with endothelial lysis or occlusive hyperplasia. The graft then becomes escharified and sloughs off as a black, hard scab. The concomitant occurrence of degenerative changes appearing in both epithelial and endothelial cells of a graft, according to the authors, implies that the immunocompetent thymus-dependent cells, known as T cells, are responsible for the graft destruction. Furthermore, the restoration of vascular continuity between the graft and host vessels during the first few days following transplantation permits the entry of host T cells into the graft and subsequent recognition of transplantation antigen on the surface of epithelial and endothelial cells, leading to blast transformation and replication of the immune cells.

As reported by Guthy *et al.* (1974), in the phenomenon of intercepted vascularization the grafts undergo one of the two following courses: some grafts show good adherence to the recipient site and successful ingrowth of proliferative host endothelial cells into the deeper layers of the dermis of the graft by 4 days. However, subsequently, the new vessels fail to penetrate deeper into the graft or to form vascular connections with the preexisting graft vessels, precluding even an abortive attempt at the restoration of two-way blood circulation. On gross examination, the grafts appear pallid, with a variable intensity of cyanosis. For the following 6–11 days the grafts retain their pallor-tan appearance before becoming desquamated as a dry crust. In contrast, other grafts show a complete absence of tissue adherence to the host bed and vascularization. There is not even a temporary ingrowth of new capillaries from the host. At 48 hours after grafting, the grafts are characterized by pallor and cyanosis, grossly becoming mummified and eosinophilic, followed by drying or secondary infection.

Guthy *et al.* (1974) concluded that the events leading to intercepted vascularization and graft demise are a combination of mechanical and technical factors such as hematoma, absence of intimate graft–host junction, or surgical dressing, and bandaging errors followed by immunologic factors. Thus, combined technical and immunologic factors prevent the effective vascular anastomosis of graft and host vessels required for establishing a definitive graft vasculature with blood flow and graft survival.

Electron Microscopic Studies

Despite the wide application of electron microscopy as a means of evaluating biologic events by clinical and research authorities in other disciplines of medicine and biology, it has not been frequently used in transplantation biology.

Wiener, Spiro, and Russell, in 1964, provided new information on the ultrastructural characteristics, supplemented by histology, of skin grafts in the rabbit, with particular reference to the participation of infiltrating host cells in graft rejection. For this experiment, full-thickness skin allografts and control autografts were transplanted from the rabbit auricles to suprapannicular recipient beds on the lateral thoracic side of the animal. Comparative histologic examinations of the test and control grafts during the first 5 days after grafting indicated good graft–host coaptation and proliferation of fibrovascular tissue in the graft, with resultant formation of granulation tissue, coupled with epithelial hyperplasia and epidermal thickening in both types of grafts. According to Wiener et al. (1964), their histologic data demonstrating this sequence of morphologic events in the graft are in line with those previously reported by other investigators. As shown by electron microscopy, the graft epidermal cells appeared well-preserved, their nuclei with prominent nucleoli still large and oval, and other elements of the epidermal cells—such as intercellular bridges, tonofibrils, vesicles, or basement membrane—distinct and easily observed, similar to those seen in normal intact skin.

By histology and electron microscopy, the earliest evidence of skin allograft rejection, at 5–7 days, is the appearance of a rapid and intense infiltration of host leukocytic cells, occurring initially in the capillaries of the graft dermis. These cells rapidly progress to the more superficial dermal layers, forming perivascular aggregates and emigrating through the endothelium of the graft vessels, without damage, into the dermal tissues to the graft epidermis. Tentatively identified as mononuclear cells on the basis of their ultrastructural characteristics differentiating them from other types of host cells, the invading cells subsequently enter the expanded intercellular spaces between the epidermal cells, without penetrating or harming the cells. These events begin in the basal cell layer and spread progressively through the strata of epidermal cells almost to the stratum corneum. Despite the strong evidence by electron microscopy of an intimate relationship between the host mononuclear cells and epidermal cells for this period of 2 days, there is no convincing indication of necrosis or degenerative changes occurring in the epidermal cells. However, this interval of intimate coexistence between the two types of cells is superseded 7–9 days after grafting by progressive degeneration of the allograft epidermis. It begins in the basal cell layer and extends through to the superficial strata of epithelium in the same pattern in which the mononuclear cells, appropriately termed the graft rejection cells, invade the graft epidermis. These events are rapidly followed by dissolution of the epithelial cell surface and desquamation of the necrotic epidermis, indicating the terminal stage of the rejection process. As reported by the authors, this sequence of events, leading to the complete degeneration of the skin allografts in the rabbit, is characterized by a complete absence of hemorrhage in the connective tissue of the graft dermis, which continues to appear unaltered.

On the basis of their findings showing progressive infiltration of mononuclear cells, clearly identified by electron microscopy, in the dermal capillaries, perivascular aggregates, and finally epidermis, with consequent necrosis of the epidermis, Wiener et al. (1964) suggest the important role of invading mononuclear cells in the graft rejection by participating as immunologically competent cells. This event allows the intimate interaction of antigen and antibody between the membranal surfaces of graft epidermal and host cells or through the areas of cytoplasmic continuity between the two cells, with resultant necrosis of the epidermis. Further evidence in support of this interpretation is the finding that necrosis of the graft epidermis clearly precedes the invasion of other types of host cells in appreciable numbers into the graft dermis.

In preliminary studies with the electron microscope, a limited but nonetheless provocative observation was the possible existence of cytoplasmic bridges between infiltrating host leukocytes and tissue structures of skin allografts in rabbits (Wiener et al. 1964) and renal allografts in dogs (Kountz, Williams, Williams, Kapros, and Dempster 1963; Williams, Williams, Kountz, and Dempster 1964). However, as explained by Wiener, Pearl, Lattes, and Spiro (1969), the evidence demonstrating this phenomenon was derived from a single level of sectioning for electron microscopy and therefore not entirely conclusive. Consequently, these investigators undertook serial electron microscopy, coupled with histology, of full-thickness suprapannicular skin auto- and allografts in the mouse in order to investigate further and to substantiate the original data.

In the allografts, numerous polymorphonuclear leukocytes of host origin emigrated through the endothelium of open-wound vessels near the graft–host junction, forming areas of cytoplasmic continuity between the two cells. Structurally, these areas of cytoplasmic continuity were characterized by areas of fusion between the surface membranes of host leukocytes and vascular endothelium of skin allografts. Consistent with this important finding was the evidence that at the areas of fusion the granules observed in the cytoplasm of endothelial cells resembled those seen in the adjacent polymorphonuclear cells, becoming fewer in number with increasing distance from the site of fusion. In contrast, such a phenomenon was not observed in control skin autografts.

The observations of Wiener et al. (1969) have extended and confirmed the previous work of others who have demonstrated the presence of cytoplasmic bridges between the invading host cells and endothelial cells of the allograft. Moreover, the demonstration of granules in the graft endothelium similar in appearance to those in the host leukocytes suggests the participation of the granules in the immune mechanism of the rejection response responsible for the rejection of skin allografts. The interpretation of the authors is that the areas of fusion facilitate the transport of granules from the cytoplasm of host cells into that of graft endothelial cells. This is followed by the release of hydrolytic enzymes from the granules into the endothelial cytoplasm, causing the endothelial degeneration.

Because the subsequent experiments by Eichwald, Pay, Busath, and Smith (1976) and Eichwald and Dolberg (1977) entail the ultrastructural appearance of skin allografts transplanted to specifically sensitized mouse recipients, resulting in the accelerated second-set phenomenon reaction of rejection, hyperacute rejection, or the white graft reaction, their reviews are deferred to Chapter 7.

Experiments with Dye Injection

Despite the increasing use of histologic techniques and various other means of investigation, there have been conflicting opinions on the relationship between the blood circulation and the immune mechanisms responsible for the deterioration and demise of allografts. For instance, Medawar (1944) cited strong histologic evidence of stagnant blood and vascular disruption during the process of skin rejection in the rabbit.

On the other hand, Ham (1952) assumed from his injection experiments with India ink that pigskin allografts are destroyed because, unlike those of autografts controls, the vascular connections with the host are not restored. Somewhat similar conclusions were reached by Conway et al. (1952) employing the transparent tissue chamber (Fig. 8) in the mouse. They reported that at 1–10 days after allotransplantation multiple thromboses appear in the vessels of the host bed coincident with the failure of the generating capillaries to invade the graft; complete necrosis of the donor tissue ensues.

Because there were such conflicting viewpoints, Scothorne and McGregor (1953) tried to resolve the problem by daily intravenous injections of bromophenol blue into rabbits. The color changes seen in the auricular skin grafts were checked by serial biopsies of some grafts, as well as by extra animal recipients given India ink intravenously. From the comparative results of auto- and allografts the investigators concluded that the cessation of circulatory blood and vascular changes constitute a part of the general pattern of allogeneic rejection. Since the events occur within 24 hours after the destruction of the donor epidermis, some other factor, not the vascular breakdown, is responsible for epidermal destruction.

Egdahl and Varco (1956) provided information concerning the disappearing properties of intradermally injected fluorescein under ultraviolet illumination as an indication of the allograft vascularization and survival end points in rabbits. From 5 to 10 days after grafting, complete disappearance of the injected material from the grafts at the same rate as from normal skin is considered strong evidence of effective restoration of circulating blood and lymphatic drainage. However, starting at 10 days, the injectant is retained by the grafts for 24–48 hours or more; the observed failure of the grafts to remove fluorescein represents the end point for the graft rejection period.

Subsequently, Egdahl *et al.* (1957) applied the intradermal fluorescein test to full-thickness skin allografts in rats; they checked it by vital microscopic examinations as practiced by Taylor and Lehrfeld (1953). As reviewed previously, the authors considered the disappearance of intradermal fluorescein and the capacity to develop localized Schwartzman reactions in 50 allografts as strong evidence of effective vascularization, as shown by stereomicroscopy. When the blood flow has ceased, the rejected graft retains the injected substance.

There has been an increasing tendency in recent years to experiment with other coloring materials to study the evolution of skin allograft rejection [e.g., Disulphine Blue in the guinea pig (Teich-Alasia, Masera, Massaioli, and Massé 1961) and in the rabbit and mouse (Kohayakawa 1966) or Patent Blue V in the mouse (Avery and Hunt 1966)]. Teich-Alasia *et al.* (1961) based their findings on the rate of diffusion, intensity, and duration of the gross color in the grafts in relation to intact recipient skin after the intracardiac injection of Disulphine Blue. The course of the patterns of color occurring in the skin allografts parallels that of autografts for the first 6 days after transplantation and is confirmed by concurrent histology. The color of the autografted tissue regresses steadily until it attains the color of the surrounding host skin by the tenth day. In sharp contrast to this, allografts fail to be colored by the injected dye at 10 days, signifying complete separation between the grafts and host sites. It has been suggested by the authors that, prior to complete graft rejection, immediate coloration is associated with a richly vascularized tissue; slow coloration is associated with signs of edema and fibrillary dissociations of the connective tissue, and occasionally erythrocytic agglutination and capillary obstruction; and slowing down of the color regression is associated with thrombosis, intravasal agglutination of red cells, and perivascular hemorrhages.

In a subsequent experiment Disulphine Blue was injected by Kohayakawa (1966) into the marginal vein of the rabbit ear and into the peritoneal cavity of mice following skin transplantation. Full-thickness autografts and allografts of rabbit auricular skin, according to him, are considered viable if they are stained intensely blue 15–20 minutes after injection of the dye. Likewise, in mice, the viability of suprapannicular skin grafts is determined 30 minutes after the intraperitoneal administration. For the first two days after grafting in the two animals, autografts and allografts fail to exhibit their staining capacity with Disulphine Blue but in the subsequent time are colored as vividly and rapidly as the surrounding host tissue, usually on the third day in rabbits and on the fifth day in mice. The successful staining capacity of the grafted skin is attributed to, and depends entirely upon the complete restoration of the blood supply in the graft dermis. Compared to the normal staining and the subsequent excretory capacity of the control autografts, the allografts gradually become less stainable as the rejection proceeds. Beginning at 8–11 days after allografting in rabbits and at 9–10 days in mice, these events are correlated with the gross appearance of edema and cyanosis and with histologic findings of epidermal necrosis, breakdown of the pilosebaceous structures, and capillary disruption, accompanied by hemorrhage containing hemosiderin and hyaline degeneration of the graft subcutaneous tissue. During the next 2 days the complete failure of the grafts to stain is associated with the survival end point of grafts. It was concluded that the survival time of a graft can be more accurately determined by injecting Disulphine Blue than by observing gross appearance alone.

In the experiment by Avery and Hunt (1966), recipient mice bearing full-thickness skin iso- and allografts were injected intraperitoneally with a dye solution of Patent Blue V. Five minutes after the dye treatment and after gross inspection of the grafts to evaluate the degree of staining, the grafts were removed with adjacent host tissue in order to correlate the histology with the degree of staining. The findings indicated that, compared to the normal staining and the subsequent excretory capacity of the isografts, which are similar to those of adjacent intact host skin, the allografts are characterized by a progression from normal staining at 6 days after grafting to nonstaining by 10 days, associated with graft rejection. Avery and Hunt concluded that the dye technique is a simple, rapid, and efficient procedure for assessing the graft behavior and its survival end points without disturbing the in situ grafts.

Biochemical Studies

Using inbred strains of rats, Moore and Schayer in 1969 were the first to provide information on changes in the pattern of intracellular histamine formation that occur in full-thickness auto- and allografts of abdominal skin. Various lines of evidence from previous experiments demonstrated that changes in the pattern of intracellular histamine metabolism caused by a variety of stimulants depend on the decarboxylation of histidine by the enzymatic action of histidine decarboxylase. Thus, first gross visual inspection and touch-palpation of the transplanted skin were performed at various 24-hour intervals until 21 days after grafting. Then skin biopsies of the graft were taken for measurement of the enzymatic activity of histidine decarboxylase by the isotope dilution method and compared with those from normal rat controls. A graft is considered rejected when it manifests the gross appearance of edematous swelling coincident with hardening, discoloration, and superficial desquamation over portions of the graft surface.

Biochemical findings indicate that in autografts the two peaks in enzymatic activity of histidine decarboxylase develop at 1 and 4 days after transplantation. As reported by these investigators, the elevations are of equal magnitude and their peaks are eight times the base level of activity noted in the normal skin of control rats. During the following 4 days, the enzymatic activity in skin autografts subsides, resuming the base level of activity seen in normal rat skin by 10 days.

In allografts, the two peak elevations also arise at 1 and 4 days after grafting, but they are one-half as great as those of autografts. (It should be mentioned that no statistical analysis of the data concerning the first two peaks of the two types of grafts was presented by Moore and Schayer.) Furthermore, in comparison to allografts evaluated 24 hours after grafting, the autografts are more firmly adherent to the recipient site. Instead of returning to the base line levels of normal intact rat skin, as is described for autografts, a significant progressive increase in the activity of the enzyme arises in skin allografts, which starts at 4 days and reaches a peak 33 times the base level of normal intact skin by 10 days. At this time, 75% of the pooled total grafted area is considered as rejected by Moore and Schayer (1969) according to their rejection criteria. Thereafter, the enzymatic activity of histidine decarboxylase subsides.

The interpretation of the changes in the pattern of intracellular histamine formation is that the presence and type of graft is capable of altering the rate of activity of histidine decarboxylase. The observation of skin allografts with two peaks of increased enzymatic activity, followed by a rapid decline toward normal levels, implies that the graft acceptance and healing process may influence the rate of histamine metabolism. One difference between autografts and allografts is the occurrence of a sharp and progressive rise of enzymatic activity in the allograft over a period extending from the fourth to the tenth day after grafting. During the first few days after allografting the initial acceptance of the graft produces a pattern of enzymatic activity similar to that described in the autografts. However, in the presence of strong histocompatibility barriers between donor and recipient, the subsequent development of inflammatory and immune responses, which leads to rejection of most grafts by 10 days, is capable of stimulating a marked increase in the rate of intracellular histamine formation.

In 1971 Jasani and Lewis described the sequence of changes in the activities of six intracellular enzymes (cathepsin, acid phosphatase, lactic dehydrogenase, β-glucuronidase, glutamic oxalacetic transaminase, and glutamic pyruvic transaminase) that occur during the life span of full-thickness orthotopic skin grafts made on hind limbs of rabbits. In addition, the concentrations of the same six enzymes were measured in the supernatant and cell pellets of the lymph, which was collected and pooled from the femoral lymphatics at various time intervals after operative procedures. No significant histologic nor histochemical differences could be ascertained between the control autografts and the test allografts during the first 5 days after transplantation. During this period the grafts changed from pale blue to bright pink, turned swollen and soft, and contained a mild inflammatory exudate consisting mostly of polymorphonuclear cells and extravasated erythrocytes.

Thereafter the sequence of events in the test grafts diverged from that in the control grafts. While the autografts gradually resumed the pale pink hue of normal skin, with a progressive subsidence of the edema and the inflammatory reaction, the allografts acquired a firm consistency, showed a significantly increased inflammatory infiltration of mononuclear or lymphocytic cells, and assumed a dull blue color. At the first sign of rejection the foreign grafts exhibited a blotchy purple appearance due to hemorrhagic necrosis, rapidly followed by widespread tissue necrosis and the eventual shedding of a hard black scab.

Jasani and Lewis (1971) injected Evans blue into the animal jugular vein and performed histologic examinations. Based on their results, they suggested that the course of vascular events, together with sequential changes in the epidermal, follicular, and dermal cells, conforms in general outline to that previously described by Medawar (1944).

A comparison of the lymph collected from the hind limbs bearing either autografts or allografts showed that the rate of lymph flow is substantially increased during the first 5 days after transplantation. Subsequently, the flow decreases to normal levels with autografts but remains significantly elevated with allografts. Under similar experimental conditions, biochemical evaluations of the supernatant of lymph show a close similarity between the results with autografts and allografts during the first 5 days after grafting. At this time there is an increase in the concentrations of cathepsin, acid phosphatase, glutamic oxalacetic transaminase, and glutamic pyruvic transaminase, whereas the activities of lactic dehydrogenase and β-glucuronidase remain unchanged. In the experiments with autografts the early increase in the activities of these four enzymes is soon followed by a return to normal levels, similar to those seen in the contralateral hind limbs without grafts. In contrast, in allografts, further increases are found in the activities of these four enzymes as well as those of the other two enzymes, lactic dehydrogenase and β-glucuronidase. Thus, according to Jasani and Lewis (1971), the surgical trauma of transplantation, not the specific properties of a skin graft, is responsible for the initial enzymatic changes.

In the cell pellets of the lymph obtained from the limbs the concentrations of all six enzymes do not change with either the autografts or allografts during the first 5 days after transplantation but then increase only with the latter. Since these enzymatic increases are not clearly correlated with the mean lymphocyte count in lymph (which can be compared to the count in lymph from nonoperated contralateral limbs), it has been suggested that some of the lymphocytes are stimulated to contain higher levels of enzyme concentrations.

Furthermore, other experimental lines of biochemical evidence demonstrate that, in general outline, the sequential patterns of all six enzymes studied in the donor skin and its host site do not parallel those in lymph but instead are governed mainly by the cellular events peculiar to the two tissues as well as by the developing immune responses associated with allograft rejection. Comparative observations show no substantial differences in the rate of progress, intensity, and duration of the enzymatic events between the autografts and allografts until the sixth day after transplantation. Starting on the third day and ending at 6 days, the activities of acid phosphatase, lactic dehydrogenase, β-glucuronidase, and cathepsin in the upper layers of a skin graft steadily increase 200–300%. These changes are said to correlate with the microscopic evidence of epithelial and fibrocytic hyperplasia, increased vascularity, and inflammatory response. On the other hand, the glutamic oxalacetic transaminase and glutamic pyruvic transaminase activities remain relatively stationary. In autografts, after the sixth day the activity of acid phosphatase, associated with an increased differentiation of the epithelial and follicular cells, continues to intensify, while those of lactic dehydrogenase, β-glucuronidase, and cathepsin, reflecting a progressive decline of inflammation, decrease. The activities of glutamic oxalacetic transaminase and glutamic pyruvic transaminase, however, remain persistently unaffected. In allografts the activities of lactic dehydrogenase, β-glucuronidase, and cathepsin continue to increase considerably more than in the autografts and in the supernatant lymph; the maximum levels are reached by day 9, about the same time as the graft is breaking down. On the other hand, the concentrations of acid phosphatase, glutamic oxalacetic transaminase, and glutaminic pyruvic transaminase remain low.

In the host bed tissue the activities of all six enzymes increase steadily during the first 3 days, these changes occurring concomitantly with the increased vascularity and inflammatory reaction. Thereafter, the activities of glutamic oxalacetic transaminase and glutamic pyruvic transaminase progressively return to normal levels, while the levels of the other four enzymes continue to increase. An obvious and persistent difference between auto- and allografts is the considerably higher enzymatic activities of β-glucuronidase and lactic dehydrogenase that occur in the tissue of the allograft bed.

Based on their biochemical findings, Jasani and Lewis (1971) concluded that the lack of lymph draining from allografts is responsible for the small magnitude of increases in the enzymatic activities of lymph at the time of and after allograft breakdown. The increase appears to occur in response to the fact that activated small lymphocytes infiltrate the graft bed and junctional tissue and then undergo necrosis. In addition, the restoration of lymphatic continuity between the graft and its host site is not a prerequisite for rejection.

Histochemical Studies

Scothorne and Tough (1952) and Scothorne and Scothorne (1953) focused attention on the possibility of using histochemical tests to evaluate the behavior and fate of the donor skin. The experiments were designed to define quantitative changes in the content of glycogen and ribonucleic acid as indicators of carbohydrate and protein metabolism, respectively, in the human pinch grafts. The results indicated that, during the latent period before the inception of the allograft rejection response, the course of the changes in the concentrations of these substances in allografts is comparable to that in autografts. However, at the time of allograft rejection, 10–15 days after transplantation, ribonucleic acid disappears. This event is in sharp contrast to the progressive return of cytoplasmic ribonucleic acid to normal levels in autografts. It would seem therefore, as suggested by Scothorne and Tough (1952), that cytoplasmic ribonucleoprotein plays an important role in the mechanism of graft destruction by acting as one of the antigens participating in the development of transplantation immunity.

With regard to the epidermal glycogen, the chain of reactions in carbohydrate metabolism is similar in the auto- and allografts until the rejection episode of the latter. However, in contrast to the complete disappearance of ribonucleic acid at 10–15 days, some of the surface epithelial cells still contain glycogen, although in variable amounts, despite the advanced stages of epidermal deterioration. According to the authors, the causative factors for the persistence of glycogen within the disrupted epidermis are not clear.

Because the histochemical experiments by Arguedas and Pérez-Tamayo (1958) in the rat focus attention on the patterns of wound healing, proliferation and deposition of collagen, fibroblastic reaction, and vascular activity in the recipient bed of skin grafts, they will not be reviewed. Subsequent studies involving the histochemical properties of grafted skin were reported by De Stefano (1959), who used rabbits, and by Donaldson, Payne, and Hershey (1960), who used guinea pigs. In view of the fact that these two studies, which describe the histochemical appearance of the enzymes alkaline phosphatase and succinic dehydrogenase, respectively, entailed the application of refrigerated skin, their reviews are deferred to Chapter 6.

Thompson (1962) provided new information on the histochemical activities and distribution of succinic dehydrogenase and protein-bound sulfhydryl groups in full-thickness skin grafts in the rat. He substantiated his findings with histologic studies. He found that, compared to the nearly normal conditions of intact skin in control autografts, the allografts are characterized by lymphocytic infiltration from the host site 3 days after transplantation. This event is rapidly followed by changes in the pattern of succinic dehydrogenase activity, which disappears from localized accumulations of epidermal cells by 4.5 days. At 5.5 days, sparsely scattered epidermal cells are necrotic, accompanied by a complete loss of the enzyme and an apparent increase in the concentration of sulfhydryl groups. Widespread cellular breakdown and severe edema are the prominent features noted in the allograft at 7 days. By the tenth day most grafts are completely rejected. Based on his observations that the early changes in the content and distribution of epithelial succinic dehydrogenase herald the graft destruction, it was suggested by Thompson that the mitochondrion, which is the site of the enzyme, plays an important role in the rejection mechanism.

After the work of Scothorne and Tough in 1952, no attempts were made to determine the vascular events in the graft by means of histochemical methods until the report, a decade later, of Converse and Ballantyne (1962) (see page 25). In the rat, biopsies of grafts with their adjacent host skin were obtained for enzyme histochemical analysis immediately after gross and stereomicroscopic inspection of the graft at predetermined time intervals. According to Converse and Ballantyne (1962) and Ballantyne, Cascarano, and Converse (1964), one early metabolic difference between auto- and allografts is the presence of a leukocytic infiltration in the allografts at 4 days. In sharp contrast to the relatively stable conditions in the autografts, there is a rapid progressive loss of diaphorase activity in the blood vessels of the allografts when undergoing the process of rejection. At the time when blood stagnation, thromboses, and hemorrhages occur in the allograft, as evidenced by in vivo stereomicroscopy, the enzymatic activity in the graft blood system has completely disappeared and the endothelial walls can no longer be discerned (Fig. 16f and h).

In addition, the initial decline of the diaphorase activity in the vessels occurs within 10–16 hours before stereomicroscopy can demonstrate the onset of the immunologic response; the deterioration of the vessels results before the cessation of hemal flow. The diminution of the enzyme activity in the vessels during the rejection period also precedes the decline in the enzymatic activity of the graft epidermis and pilosebaceous structures (Fig. 16g). For these reasons, the authors concluded that the graft vessels are affected by the immune system of the host before the epidermis and hair follicles are affected.

A careful and thorough series of histochemical studies on the metabolic activities of two oxidative and several hydrolytic enzymes in split-thickness grafts was next reported by Wolff and Schellander (1966b). These workers used unrelated male and female pigs. They confirmed the histochemical results of Converse and Ballantyne (1962) in the rat with regard to DPN diaphorase activity in allografts (Fig. 36a). In addition, they found that the reduction of other enzymatic activities (Fig. 36b) within the graft vasculature, with the exception of acid and alkaline phosphastase reactions, precedes the allograft reaction. While agreeing with Converse and Ballantyne regarding the rapid progressive loss of diaphorase activity in the vascular system before it occurs in other tissue elements of the transplant, Wolff and Schellander suggested that the rejection is not due solely to the breakdown

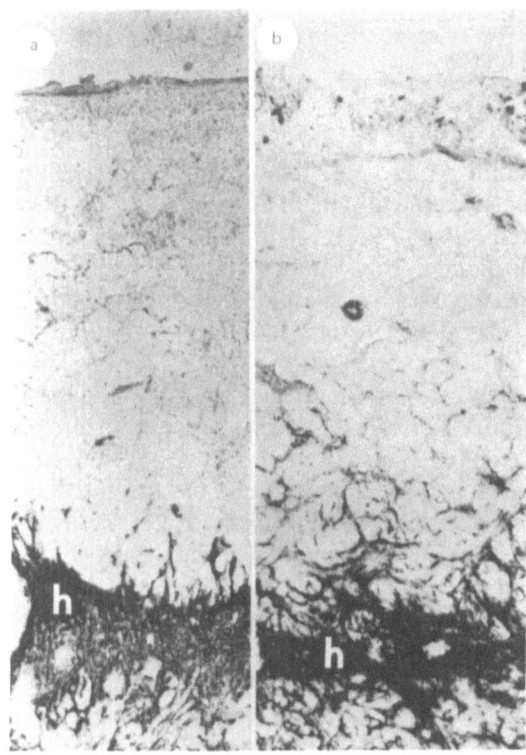

Fig. 36 a and b. Histochemical study of enzymatic activity in porcine grafts. **a.** DPN diaphorase activity in an allograft after 7 days. The graft shows no enzymatic activity with the exception of a few connective tissue cells in its lowermost portions. The healing zone *(h)* connecting the graft *(top)* and the recipient tissue *(bottom)* displays heavy formazan deposits. **b.** Aminopeptidase activity in an allograft after 8 days. Residual activity is still present in the deep portions of the graft; the upper parts of the tissue are free of enzymatic reactions. The healing zone *(h)* is strongly positive. ×45. Wolff and Schellander (1966) J. Invest. Dermatol. 46:213, © (1966) The Williams & Wilkins Co., Baltimore.

of the blood vessels by the immune response of the host, but rather to direct damage of the other graft tissues independently of the blood circulation. However, the authors decided that the reduction of most of the various enzymatic activities is the result of the effects of the rejection process on cellular function. Both Converse and Ballantyne (1962) and Wolff and Schellander (1966b) expressed similar viewpoints that the decline of metabolic activity in the allogeneic tissues constitutes an early and irreversible sign of the impending immune reaction.

A later histochemical experiment concerned with the leucine-aminopeptidase (LAP) activity in association with skin rejection was conducted by Vaino and Alfthan (1969) working with inbred and outbred guinea pigs. No appreciable difference in the enzymatic pattern of the grafted skin was noted between the groups of outbred and control inbred recipients. Likewise, the LAP reaction in other laboratory animals (rats and hamsters) exhibited a similar pattern, although quantitatively different, when compared with that in the guinea pig. Thus, from a practical standpoint, it was concluded that this enzyme histochemical method is not an effective criterion of the graft condition and survival end points.

Transparent Tissue Chamber Studies

Direct Observation of Skin Grafts In Situ

For the purpose of direct microscopic observations of living tissue cells in situ over long periods of time, Sandison, in 1924, first designed a transparent tissue chamber that could be placed on the auricle of a rabbit. Because there were certain physiologic problems in the early chambers, the use of the transparent chamber technique did not excite much interest until Algire (1943a) successfully adapted the apparatus to the mouse by using a dorsal fold of skin. Encouraged by the usefulness of this technique as a tool in the study of transplanted tumors in vivo in the mouse, Algire and Legallais (1949) made several changes in the design of the mouse transparent chamber to overcome defects in the previous chambers. In 1951, Conway, Joslin, and Stark first applied the principle of the transparent tissue chamber to skin grafts, with particular attention to technical considerations and modifications of the procedures designed by Algire and Legallais. Later, Conway, Stark, and Joslin (1951) reported their findings on the early physiologic phases of circulation in full-thickness autografts (see pages 2 and 14).

In 1952, Conway, Joslin, Rees, and Stark refined the chamber technique (Fig. 8) by means of a copper wire frame of traction splint developed by Joslin (1952) for the physical support of the dorsal skin fold. They reported that 1–10 days after grafting allogeneic skin fails to become vascularized, coincident with increased vascularity and multiple thromboses within the vessels in the host bed, followed by complete graft necrosis. These results have been suggested as an explanation of the allograft rejection. However, stereomicroscopic studies by Taylor and Lehrfeld (1953) showed that allografts in the rat, like control autografts, are successfully vascularized prior to the rejection reaction; their findings showing revascularization of autografts and allografts were confirmed in man by Converse and Rapaport (1956). After the administration of India ink or bromophenol into the vascular system of rabbits, Scothorne and McGregor (1953) also found evidence of effective vascularization in allografts.

Further evidence of the effective restoration of blood circulation in allografts was reported by Edgerton and Edgerton (1955). They used a rather more elaborate modification of the Algire-Legallais tissue chamber in which a "two-sided chamber" was included to serve to improve visual observation. Briefly, the authors found that the mouse skin allografts, like the autograft controls, become pink grossly and well vascularized microscopically in the first 9–10 days after surgery. However, within the next 24 hours—unlike autografts, which remain consistently stable—the circulation in the allografts becomes sluggish, the blood vessels dilate, and the foreign tissue begins to deteriorate; meanwhile the vascular activity in the host bed under the grafts increases without any evidence of thrombosis. It was concluded by the investigators that the graft breakdown is not the outcome of a nutritional death due to circulatory failure.

In order to reinvestigate the mechanism of the rejection response under more appropriate physiologic conditions, with an emphasis on better visual evaluations of grafts in situ, Edgerton, Peterson, and Edgerton (1957) made further adjustments in the design of their mouse window chamber by incorporating modifications of the original Joslin splint and of their previous two-sided chamber (Fig. 37). Improved visibility for serial observations within the resultant chamber was facilitated by means of an optical glass disc inserted onto the back side of the graft bed, permitting direct view of the graft undersurface. The microscopic findings, confirmed by the gross appearance of untreated orthotopic control grafts, indicate that the onset of and the restoration of blood supply, followed by other vascular changes during the first 7 days after grafting, including the rate and extent of vascularization, are similar in the autografts and allografts. However, unlike the permanent persistence of the autografts, with the allografts, usually on the eighth day, a definite increase in the caliber and the number of blood vessels, accompanied by hyperemia, is seen in the recipient bed; this event is rapidly followed by a sudden reduction in the caliber of the graft vessels concomitant with a slowing of the blood flow rate. According to the findings of Edgerton et al. (1957) with the chamber system, the survival time for 200 allografts is 9 days plus or minus 24 hours. At no time was there any evidence of thrombosis within the vessels of the host site.

Stimulated by the criticisms of Scothorne and McGregor (1953) and Taylor and Lehrfeld (1953), as well as by the encouraging findings of Edgerton and Edgerton (1955) and Edgerton et al. (1957) using the mouse chamber technique, Conway, Griffith, Shannon, and Findley (1957) and Conway, Sedar, and Shannon (1957) made technical refinements in their chamber system (Fig. 9). They incorporated improvements in the design of the copper wire splint and chamber assembly by means of a Saran plastic window preparation. The authors then found evidence of active blood circulation in the allografts of mouse skin between 3 and 6 days after grafting. As for the sequence of vascular events prior to and during the rejection period, Conway, Griffith, Shannon, and Findley (1957) confirmed the observations of Edgerton et al. (1955) in the mouse, as well as the stereomicroscopic observations of Taylor and Lehrfeld (1953) in the rat and Converse and Rapaport (1956) in man.

Studies of the Microvasculature

The transparent tissue chamber has been frequently used as an experimental model for observing in vivo vascular changes in skin grafts, with particular attention to the revascularization process. However, it was not until 1970 that Zarem and Dimitrievich employed the chamber technique for assessing

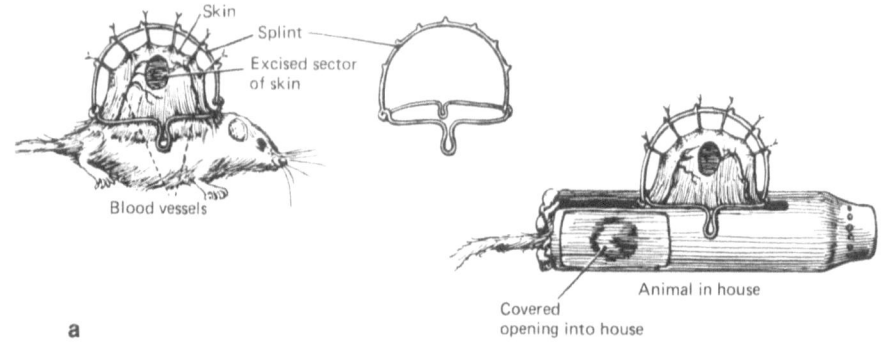

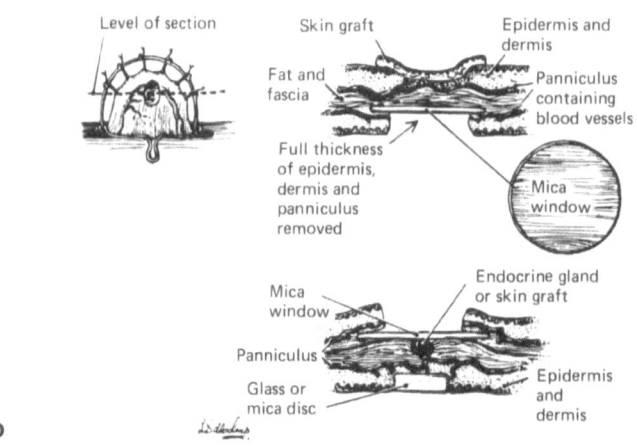

Fig. 37 a and b. Transparent mouse chamber. **a.** Arrangement of copper wire splint. A fold of dorsal skin is held up by means of a half-circle splint. Tantalum or stainless steel sutures are used to secure the skin fold to the splint. The two side arms or "outriggers" stabilize the splint in the vertical position. *Bottom:* the mouse is shown in the brass holder used for microscopic viewing. A strip of cellophane (Scotch) tape covers an opening in the cylinder through which a leg may be drawn for various injections. **b.** Cross sections of transparent mouse chambers. *Upper left:* level of cross sections *(broken line)* shown. *Top:* the recent physiologic type of chamber that may be used to study skin grafts. Note that, except for the graft itself, light need be transmitted only through one layer of fascia and one layer of blood vessels. The mica or glass window is held in place simply by overlapping skin edges. In this way the trauma from sutures is avoided. *Bottom:* details of the type of chamber employed in the study of grafts other than skin. The epidermis and dermis have been removed from both surfaces of the skin fold, with great care having been taken to spare the vessels of the panniculus carnosus on the back "side" of the chamber. Edgerton, Peterson, and Edgerton (1957) Arch. Surg. 74:238, © 1957, American Medical Association.

the microvasculature within full-thickness mouse allografts before and during the rejection period. This experiment was designed to compare skin allografts in normal untreated recipient mice serving as controls with those in mice given Imuran.

The findings indicated that in normal control allografts there is a progressive differentiation of the dilated vessels into a mature complex of arteries, capillaries, and venules within 5–8 days after grafting. By 8 and 10 days 65% and 80% of the grafts, respectively, shows an intense cellular inflammatory infiltrate. Endothelial swelling first noted in the microvasculature of a few allografts at 7 days is rapidly followed, usually within 24–48 hours, by white cells rolling along and sticking to the vessel wall. However, despite the early evidence of white cell rolling and adherence to the vessel wall in association with endothelial swelling, persistent white blood cell sticking and occlusion of the small vessels by white blood cell plugs does not develop in most grafts until day 11. Swelling of the endothelium within the graft microvasculature is considered a sign of vascular damage mediated by inflammatory cells, necessary for the subsequent sticking together of white blood cells. The appearance of endothelial swelling coincident with in vivo evidence of white blood cell plugs compromising the vascular lumen has been interpreted by Zarem and Dimitrievich (1970) as the principal factor responsible for the obstruction of vessels and complete cessation of blood flow through the microvasculature in the majority of allografts by day 13. Of particular importance is the finding that during the vascular changes leading to the graft breakdown rouleaux formation and red cell thrombi do not appear to participate in causing the obstruction.

Radioisotope and Autoradiographic Studies

Another experimental approach to the problem of elucidating the role of vascular and circulatory changes in allograft breakdown has been through the use of radioactive materials. It was introduced by Ohmori and Kurata in 1960. Ten minutes after intravenous injections of a crystalloid ^{32}P solution into rabbits, graft biopsies were taken and the levels of radioactivity were measured with a Geiger-Müller counter. The measurements of the transfer rates of the isotopes, reflecting the circulatory condition in the autografts and allografts, showed that on the sixth day the circulation in the allografts, while still functional, is not as active as that in the autografts. In the allograft, the circulation diminishes rapidly until it ceases completely on day 9, whereas in autografts the blood flow improves, becoming normal by day 20. These observations of circulatory events, as assessed by the isotope technique, were confirmed by concurrent histology. The diminution of blood flow in the allogeneic graft is characterized by histologic evidence of thrombotic capillaries that increase in severity with the progressive decrease in the rate of blood circulation. Ohmori and Kurata (1960) considered the cessation of blood flow, the result of an antigen–antibody reaction, to be an important factor in the failure of the grafts to survive, but the actual causal factors could not be clearly defined.

Similar results have been obtained in rabbits by Pihl and Weiber (1963), who also applied the radioisotope technique with ^{32}P (Fig. 22). Although there is empirical evidence that the reduction in the impulse frequency of injected isotopes is associated with the graft degeneration, no theory has been advanced by the authors to explain the appearance of congestion, thrombosis, and hemorrhage in the grafts undergoing rejection.

Walker and Goldman (1963) used tritiated thymidine autoradiography in the mouse. They reported on the participation by infiltrative leukocytes in allograft rejection and the responses of the graft epithelium, fibroblasts, and endothelium to the alien environment. The experiment entails injections of tritiated thymidine into the host mice either before or after transplantation of full-thickness orthotopic grafts. The animals are killed at various time intervals for fluid emulsion autoradiography of the grafted area. Histologic observations showing increased fibroblast and endothelial populations at the base of skin grafts appear to be well correlated with the increased uptake of the radioactive isotope by fibroblasts and endothelial cells. The number of proliferating fibroblasts increases rapidly with time until a layer of these cells forms under the grafted skin; it is particularly more prominent in mice bearing allografts. In addition, large numbers of labeled leukocytes migrate into the allografts from the blood, while only a few of these cells are found in the isografts. Walker and Goldmann (1963) discussed the possible role of these cells in the allograft rejection mechanism but did not make any definite conclusions.

In order to gain further insight into the process of antigen recognition by which the information on histocompatibility differences is transmitted between the graft and its host, Lambert and Frank (1967) undertook studies of skin grafts labeled with tritiated thymidine in rabbits (Fig. 38a and b). Autoradiographs of auricular skin grafts, tagged by the radioactive isotope injected intravenously into the recipient animal, show a higher level of proliferation of capillary endothelial cells and fibroblasts at the site of an allograft than that of an autograft; this event appears as early as the first day after grafting. In addition to this, tagged nuclear components released from the graft epithelial cells are transferred and incorporated into nuclei of host cells in the surrounding tissue (Fig. 38c and d). The authors considered these findings strong experimental evidence that allogeneic differences can be locally recognized and responded to almost immediately after tissue transplantation. In addition to providing information on histocompatibility differences by surface contact effect, the endothelial cells and fibroblasts serve a vital role in graft revascularization and in healing.

Comparison Between Conventional and Immediately Vascularized Allografts

In order to achieve an immediate vascularization of grafted skin in the rat, Gruber, Kaplan, and Lucas (1974) devised a transplantation model in which a vascular flap of full-thickness skin removed from the donor's abdomen was anastomosed to the recipient femoral vessels by microvascular techniques. Some of the vascularized skin flaps were rendered alymphatic by inserting

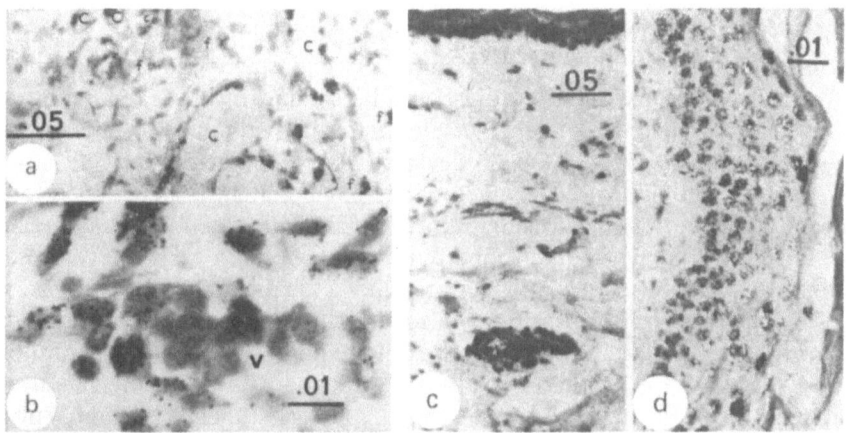

Fig. 38 a and b. Nuclear labeling in relation to skin grafts (scales represent fractions of a millimeter). **a.** Autoradiograph of a 46-hour allograft labeled by tritiated thymidine given intravenously to the host. Labeled capillary endothelial cells and fibroblasts are demonstrated at the graft–host interface. The vasculature had been injected with a radiopaque mass (Micropaque) before the ear was fixed, allowing easy recognition of the somewhat distended fine vessels. c, capillary; f, fibroblast. **b.** Autoradiograph of host cells deep in the bed of a 4-day allograft labeled prior to transfer. A small vessel (v) containing erythrocytes is lined by labeled endothelial cells, one of which is in mitosis. The remaining labeled cells are fibroblasts. All labels in this panel are derived from the nuclei of labeled graft cells. (Graft and bed were infiltrated with nonradioactive thymidine.)

c and d. Autoradiographs of skin labeled before transplantation (scales represent fractions of a millimeter). **c.** Skin immediately before grafting. Silver grains, considerably in excess of background density, can be seen adjacent to the heavily labeled hair follicle and basal layer of the epidermis, suggesting that some labeled material may have been released by these cells. **d.** Epithelium of the same skin 7 days after transplantation as an allograft. The initial heavy labeling of the basal cells has not interfered with the usual extensive proliferation of the epithelial cells. Lambert and Frank (1967) Science 155 (6 Jan.):99, © 1967 by the American Association for the Advancement of Science.

between the graft and its bed a silicone sheet with a central opening for the vascular stalk. Daily gross observations and serial histologic examinations were done to assess the graft behavior and survival times; complete mummification, necrosis, or hemic extravasation within the donor tissue was considered a diagnostic indication of graft rejection.

Despite the immediate vascularization of allogeneic skin flaps achieved by microvascular anastomoses, the survival time was not significantly different from that of conventional allografts. It was concluded that the time of rejection is not correlated with the rate of vascularization nor the condition of graft vascularity. The results of this experiment also suggest that ischemia is not an important factor since the allograft survival time was not enhanced by eliminating ischemia. Even when the vascularized skin flap was made alymphatic at transplantation, there was no significant improvement in survival time as compared to that of either the conventional or immediately vascularized allografts. This observation has been interpreted as strong circumstantial evidence that, whereas the development of heightened resistance to conventional skin allografts is primarily provided by the lymphatic vessels, under experimental conditions the hosts can be effectively sensitized by the exposure to antigenic stimuli via the direct venous connections alone. The relatively long periods needed for host sensitization to skin after transplantation may simply reflect the time required for new growth of blood and lymphatic vessels, thereby permitting adequate entry of antigen into the recipient or of host cells into the graft (Converse, Ballantyne, and Woisky 1958; McKhann and Berrian 1959b; Henry and Dammin 1962; Barker and Billingham 1968; Billingham and Barker 1969).

The results of Gruber et al. (1974), however, do not agree qualitatively with those of Barker and Billingham (1968), who showed that, in the guinea pig, vascularized skin flaps deprived of lymphatic connections long outlive conventional skin allografts despite the vascular continuity between the donor tissue and its host. Barker and Billingham (1968) concluded that with orthotopic allografts of skin intact efferent drainage is an essential prerequisite for sensitization of the host.

Further efforts were made by Wustrack, Gruber, and Lucas in 1975 to establish the role of blood and lymphatic vessels in mediating sensitization of the host by skin allografts. They used four skin grafting techniques (Fig. 39) that differed in vascular and lymphatic reconstitution rates. For the first skin grafting model in the rat, the investigators followed a technique modified from that of Billingham and Medawar (1951) for preparing conventional full-thickness allografts and control isografts in which the draining lymphatics are immediately reconstituted (delayed vascular–immediate lymphatic reconstitution, DV-IL). For the second grafting model (delayed vascular–delayed lymphatic reconstitution, DV-DL), they placed skin grafts on a vascular flap of skin rendered alymphatic by inserting between the flap and its bed a silicone sheet with a central hole for the vascular stalk, following

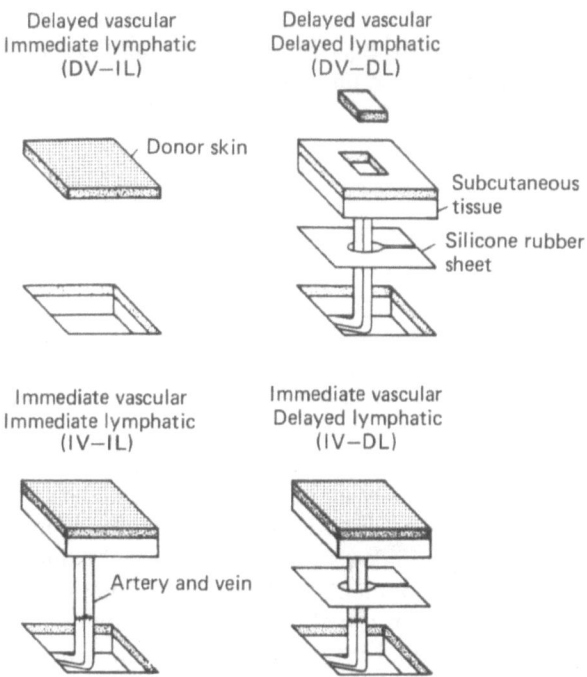

Delayed vascular
Immediate lymphatic
(DV–IL)

Delayed vascular
Delayed lymphatic
(DV–DL)

Donor skin

Subcutaneous tissue

Silicone rubber sheet

Immediate vascular
Immediate lymphatic
(IV–IL)

Immediate vascular
Delayed lymphatic
(IV–DL)

Artery and vein

Fig. 39. Four skin graft models differing in rates of vascular and lymphatic reconstitution. Wustrack, Gruber, and Lucas (1975) Transplantation 19:156, © (1975) The Williams & Wilkins Co., Baltimore.

the microvascular technique of Barker and Billingham (1968) (described in more detail on page xvi). The other two grafting models used were the microvascular anastomosis of a composite skin flap with effective lymphatic drainage (immediate vascular–immediate lymphatic reconstitution, IV-IL) and an alymphatic vascular flap of skin (immediate vascular–delayed lymphatic reconstitution, IV-DL). The immediately vascularized skin flaps were prepared according to the microvascular technique of Strauch and Murray (1967). The IV-DL grafts differed in that the normal lymphatic drainage was interrupted by a silicone sheet interposed between the graft and host bed.

On the basis of gross observations confirmed by occasional histology and angiography, Wustrack and associates (1975) stated that in the rat allografts transplanted by a conventional grafting technique (DV-IL), onto immediately vascularized flaps (IV-IL), or onto alymphatic vascularized flaps (IV-DL) demonstrate similar mean survival times of 7.8 days. In contrast, grafts placed on a vascular flap of skin with interrupted lymphatic drainage (DV-DL) enjoy prolonged survival, doubling the mean time to 15.6 days. It was concluded that either intact lymphatic drainage or vascular connection between graft and host is adequate and both are equally effective in sensitizing the host with antigenic material from the graft. If both draining lymphatics and vascular contact are interrupted (DV-DL), the grafts survive longer because there is interference with the afferent phase of the sensitizing antigens from the grafts. These findings also agree with those of Tilney and Gowans (1971) in skin allografts transplanted to the alymphatic vascular flap of host skin in the rat.

Other Experimental Studies

Attempts were made by Ljungqvist and Almgård (1966) to define the behavior and fate of circular skin auto- and allografts placed on the rabbit auricles by means of a combined stereomicroangiographic and histologic technique (Fig. 15a and b), as described in more detail on page 24. Their data show no difference in vascularity between the two types of grafts during the developmental stage of graft vascularization. This conformity ends when the allografts are rejected, as evidenced by the avascular areas of necrosis alternating with remaining viable tissue containing thrombi in the thin-walled and dilated vessels. These findings led Ljungqvist and Almgård to conclude that rejection and the development of necrosis could not be attributed to the failure of revascularization in the allografts, as originally assumed by Conway *et al.* (1952). They found it difficult to ascertain whether the changes noted in the established graft vasculature were responsible for the allograft breakdown.

With an approach somewhat similar to stereomicroscopy, Nilsson, Obel, and Schantz (1971), working with dogs, developed a new in vivo diagnostic assay method for assessing the behavior and survival time of skin grafts transplanted to the perichondrial surface on the dorsum of recipient ears. In this technique the grafts are transilluminated by a light source behind the ventral aspect of the auricles and the light permeability of the grafts is measured with a photometer. These findings are then correlated with the results of histologic examinations of the grafts.

The increase in the light permeability of both autografts and allografts during the first 5 days after grafting is reflected by histologic evidence of nonspecific inflammatory changes, edema, and mild leukocytic infiltration at the graft periphery. Starting at 7 or 8 days there is a sudden reduction of the light permeability of the allografts; upon microscopic examination, this stage is generally characterized by massive lymphocytic and polymorphonuclear infiltration (Fig. 40a) in addition to the diffuse hemorrhages and degenerative processes of the graft epithelium and dermis (Fig. 40b). Furthermore, by either histology or light permeability, there are no basic differences between the split-thickness skin grafts and the full-thickness grafts undergoing the reaction of immune rejection. Nilsson and associates (1971) recommend the use of their light measurement technique as a sensitive and simple indicator of graft survival time resulting from the use of immunosuppressive measures.

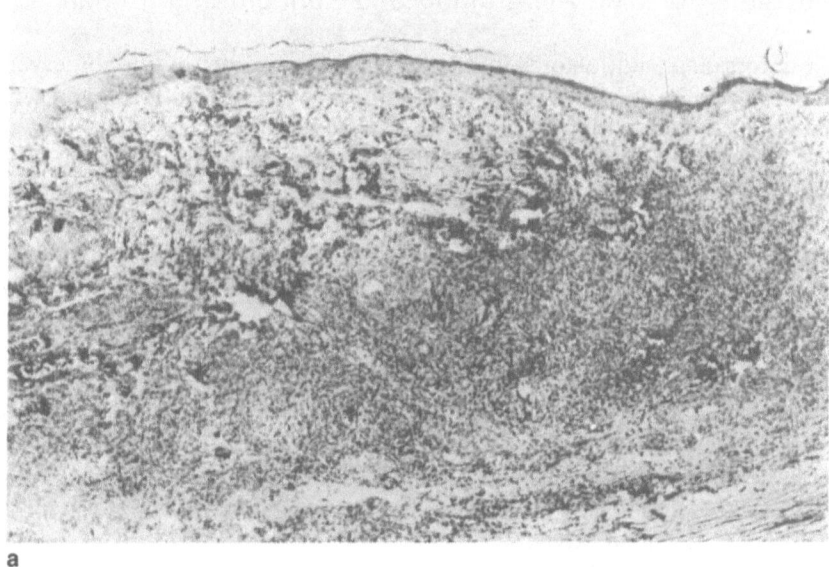

a

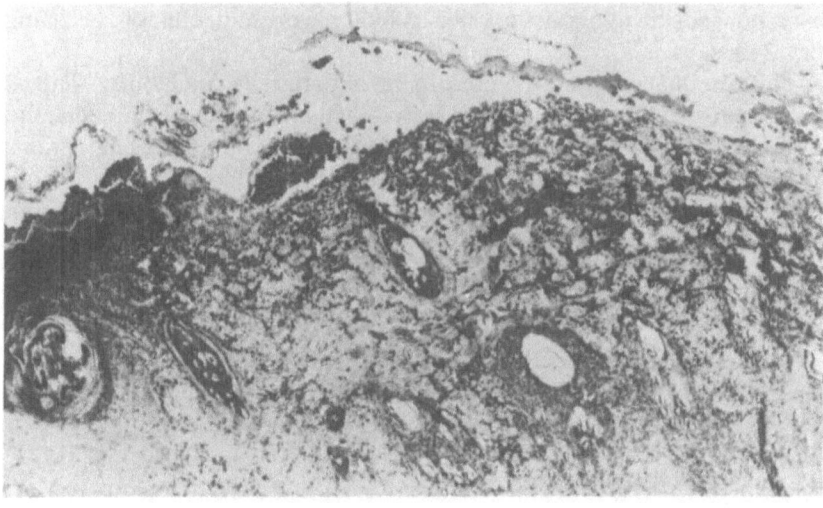

b

Fig. 40 a and b.   Histologic sections demonstrating allograft rejection. **a.** Histologic rejection stage 3. Massive infiltration by lymphocytes, histiocytes, polymorphonuclear leukocytes, and plasma cells of the graft border zone. H & E. ×50. **b.** Histologic rejection stage 4. Severe necrobiotic and necrotic changes in the epithelium and the corium of the graft with diffuse hemorrhages and infiltration by lymphocytes and polymorphonuclear leukocytes. H & E. ×50. Nilsson, Obel, and Schantz (1971) Acta Chir. Scand. 137:315.

Indications for Skin Allografting and Xenografting in Man

Free autotransplantation of skin is widely used in reconstructive surgery and usually produces excellent results under normal conditions. However, when a patient has a loss of full-thickness skin coverage exceeding 30% of the body surface due to burns or mechanical trauma, autografts are often not available in sufficient quantity or could only be obtained at considerable disadvantage, risk, or discomfort to the patient, particularly in infants or children (Woodruff 1960; Bromberg and Song 1966; State and Peter 1974). Temporary coverage can be obtained by means of skin allografts from volunteers, recently deceased patients, or the patient's relatives and friends and is often a life-saving measure. The use of allografts prevents protein and electrolyte loss, reduces bacterial contamination and pain, and decreases body fluid and heat loss. In addition, it gives the patient a brief respite during which his general condition has the time to improve and recover. Réverdin recommended the use of skin allografts in 1872, and Brown, Fryer, Randall, and Lu (1953) advocated their use as biologic dressings for extensive burn wounds and denuded areas.

The initial vascularization of skin allografts and their ultimate immunologic rejection have already been reviewed. In order to avoid a rejection response, skin allografts applied as biologic dressings should be changed every 2–3 days.

The chief handicap in the use of skin allografts is availability. They can be obtained fresh, usually from relatives, and either used immediately or stored after rapid freezing (see Chapter 6). Large crops of allogeneic skin can also be obtained from disease-free cadavers.

As noted by Artz, Rittenbury, and Yarbrough (1972), skin allografts used as biologic dressings can serve several functions:

Clean up granulating areas prior to autografting.
Protect open wounds from water and protein loss until autografts are available.
Decrease pain at the site of an open wound.
Facilitate early motion of the affected part.
Decrease surface bacterial counts.
Cover exposed vital structures.
Enhance the growth of any underlying epithelium (questionable).

In burn patients, fortunately, the survival of skin allografts is prolonged (Rapaport and associates, 1964). Allergic responses of the delayed hypersensitivity type are also depressed by thermal injury (Casson, Solowey, Converse, and Rapaport 1966). Immunologic paralysis, antigen competition, and the change sharing of histocompatibility antigens by randomly selected unrelated individuals are probably factors accounting for these phenomena following thermal injury.

Batchelor and Hackett (1970) showed that if the HLA antigen incompatibility of any allograft donor is limited to one or less, allograft survival of 2 months or more can be expected in patients with third-degree burns involving more than 40% of the body surface area.

The technique of alternating skin auto- and allografts for obtaining skin coverage for areas of extensive skin loss, such as occur in deep burns, was proposed by Mcwlem (1952) and described by Jackson (1954). The technique has been largely replaced by the application of skin allografts under which "seeds" of autografts are placed. The technique of alternating autografts and allografts has been described by Colson, Leclerq, Gangolphe, Houot, Janvier, and Prunieras (1959), who have also studied the histology of the progressive replacement of the allografts by the autografts.

The Chinese (Burns Unit, 1973) reported remarkable improvement in survival rates following massive burns involving more than 70% of the body surface (third-degree burns exceeding 50% of the body surface area). After early debridement of the eschars, minute skin autografts were introduced through buttonholes in large sheets of cadaver skin and young white pigskin allografts which covered the burn wounds. The allografts provided favorable wound conditions for the spread and growth of the island autografts.

Skin allografts have also been recommended for coverage of second-degree burns (Miller, Switzer, Foley, and Moncrief 1967; Miller and White 1972). In addition to providing relief of pain and inhibition of evaporative and exudative water loss, skin allografts promote healing with an improved cosmetic result.

Miller (1974) has cautioned against coverage of split-thickness skin donor sites with viable skin allografts, as rejection of the latter results in conversion of the donor site from a partial-thickness to a full-thickness defect.

Summary

On the basis of essentially similar results obtained from all the various assay procedures described thus far, the orderly sequence of events that leads to the rejection reaction of skin allografts begins with round cell infiltration, occasionally accompanied by polymorphonuclear cells at the host–graft junction. It continues with widespread graft edema, progressive engorgement, and dilation of the graft vascular system with a gradually diminishing blood flow, and terminates with an inflammatory reaction, often violent in intensity, along with a complete stagnation of blood circulation, thrombosis, and rupture of the graft vasculature. Following the breakdown of the vascular walls, with extensive extravasation of blood cells, the graft undergoes hemorrhagic necrosis and eventually sloughs off as a hard dry brown or black scab, leaving a dermal pad in the recipient site. During the ensuing reparative process, the dermal pad is temporarily incorporated into the regenerating host dermis, then is slowly absorbed, and finally is replaced by scar tissue.

Although there is considerable disagreement with respect to the mechanism of the immunologic reaction in the conventional graft–host relationship by which the graft is destroyed and its relationship to the graft vascular system, a significant and characteristic feature seen in the majority of the histologic studies and other experimental and clinical diagnostic methods is the morphologic change that takes place in the vascular network immediately before changes occur in the other tissue elements of the graft (Medawar 1944, 1945; Taylor and Lehrfeld 1953; Egdahl *et al*. 1957; Converse and Ballantyne 1962; Henry *et al*. 1962; Wolff and Schellander 1966a).

There is ample evidence, accumulated from the experiments of Hall (1967), Barker and Billingham (1967, 1968), Billinghan and Barker (1969) and others, that the lymphatic vessels draining the site of skin allografts are the principal access of antigenic stimuli to the host regional lymph nodes, where the antigenic-sensitive, or immunologically competent, cells with the morphologic features of small, thymus-derived, lymphocytes are activated by the graft antigens. Following confrontation with the antigenic material, these cells settle in the regional nodes and are transformed into large pyroninophilic cells, or immunoblasts, which, in turn, rapidly proliferate into a crop of small lymphocytes. These cells, termed the derived sensitized lymphocytes or effector cells, eventually enter the blood stream via efferent lymphatic vessels and initiate the process of allograft rejection by attacking and inflicting damage on the graft target cells.

Chapter 3

Chronic Reaction Patterns of First-Set Skin Allografts

As stated in the Introduction, if a first-set allograft of skin is not rapidly and violently destroyed within 2 weeks by its host, it is capable of evoking a milder form of cellular inflammatory reaction and will show protracted survival with no evidence of incompatibility. In some instances the graft may survive permanently.

This chapter is concerned with skin allograft reactions that are characterized by a prolonged latent period of survival, preceded by a chronic tissue rejection reaction. Because there is a relative paucity of literature available on this subject, it is difficult at this time to separate distinct discrepancies in the course of morphologic and vascular events reflecting variable patterns of chronic skin allograft rejection, but an attempt at a composite description will be made.

Studies in the Hamster

According to the work of Adams, Patt, and Lutz (1956) with golden hamsters, the manifestations of chronic rejection of full-thickness skin allografts, whether interstrain or intrastrain, are loss of hair, hemorrhagic foci in the graft dermis, epidermal flaking, and gradual destruction and replacement by scar tissue. In terms of intensity and degree the altered reactivity seems more apparent in the allografts exchanged between interstrain colonies of hamsters than in those taken from intrastrain lines.

The findings of Adams *et al.* (1956) were extended and verified by Billingham and Hildemann (1958a, b) in similar animals obtained from four independent closed colonies. Beginning at 8 days after grafting and at 2–4-day intervals thereafter, the condition, viability, and survival times of full-thickness skin allografts were evaluated on the basis of the graft's outward appearance, supplemented whenever necessary by histology. It is

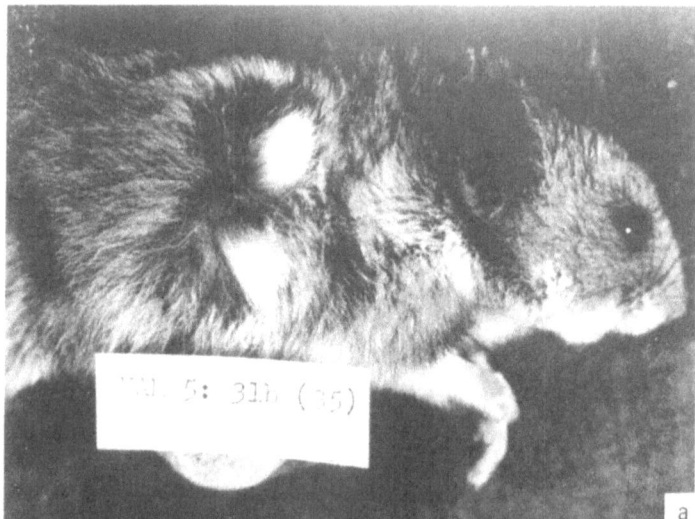

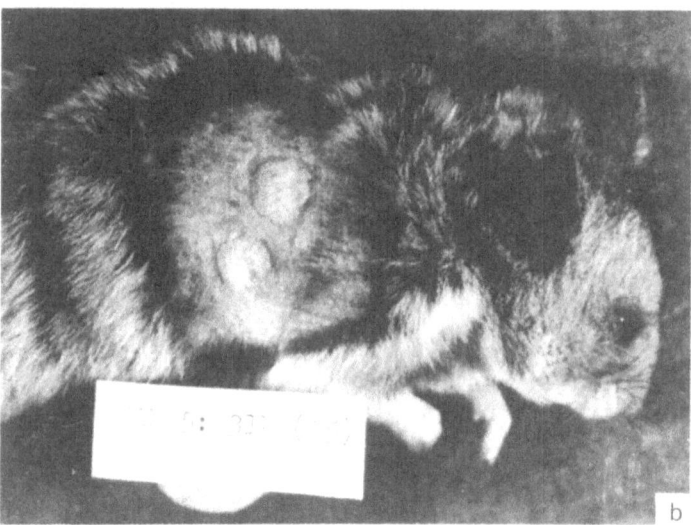

Fig. 41 a and b. Successful intercolony homografts in normal adult Syrian hamsters, MHA → LSH. **a.** Albino skin grafts on agouti host 35 days after grafting. Note dense crops of white hair with reversed orientation. **b.** The same grafts after hair has been clipped. Billingham and Hildemann (1958) Ann. N.Y. Acad. Sci. 73:676.

evident from the data that a high degree of compatibility existed in most of the allografts in which the grafting procedure was done between members of a closed hamster colony. The grafts behaved like autografts—as indicated by the resumption of the normal appearance of skin and by the regeneration of normal hair crops with reversed orientation at 30 days (Fig. 41)—and survived for at least 100 days. However, a few of the grafts eventually did become edematous and inflamed, followed by a general thinning of the hair crop, scaly exfoliation of the graft dermis, and prolonged chronic inflammatory reaction accompanied by a progressive contraction of the graft.

The existence, incidence, and nature of the immune reaction against grafted skin in this species, as characterized by variable patterns of chronic skin allograft rejection, vary from one specific closed colony of Syrian hamsters to another. For example, every recipient from the colony of LSH hamsters maintained its graft for more than 100 days without any evidence of a rejection, whereas 67% of the CB intracolony allografts survived without alteration during the same time period.

On the other hand, when the grafts were reciprocally transplanted between individuals of different hamster colonies, a much greater variability in graft behavior and survival times was observed. For example, 13 of 18 MHA colony recipient hamsters acutely rejected the grafts from CB colony hamsters within 2 weeks, while three of the remaining MHA colony animals fully accepted their CB colony grafts for at least 100 days. In contrast, all of the MHA colony recipients retained their grafts from the LSH colony for 100 days or more, but 5 of 17 LSH animals with MHA colony grafts rejected their grafts in an acute fashion within 14 days after transplantation. It is presumed that the nature of the rejection mechanisms and the survival times of skin allografts between different colonies of hamsters depend upon antigenic differences, and these in turn depend upon genetic differences between certain donor and host combinations.

Similarly, in a subsequent study using adult Syrian hamsters drawn from a closed but outbred colony, Hildemann and Walford (1960) described the existence, grossly and histologically, of the anomalous acceptance or rejection of skin allografts by the recipient animals. Of 55 animals grafted, only 4 first-set allografts underwent an acute rejection reaction, as grossly demonstrated by hemostasis, inflammation, and epithelial weakness by the end of 14 days. In contrast, the remaining 51 grafts (92.7%) persisted for periods of from 19 to more than 550 days. As stated in the Introduction, Hildemann and Walford have classified the different patterns of the delayed rejection mechanism into three categories in order of increasing survival times: (1) *rapid chronic*, with survival end points of 19–61 days (Figs. 42a and b); (2) *intermediate chronic*, with survival times ranging from 78 to over 261 days; and (3) *prolonged chronic* (Figs. 42c and d), with protracted graft survival from 307 to over 550 days.

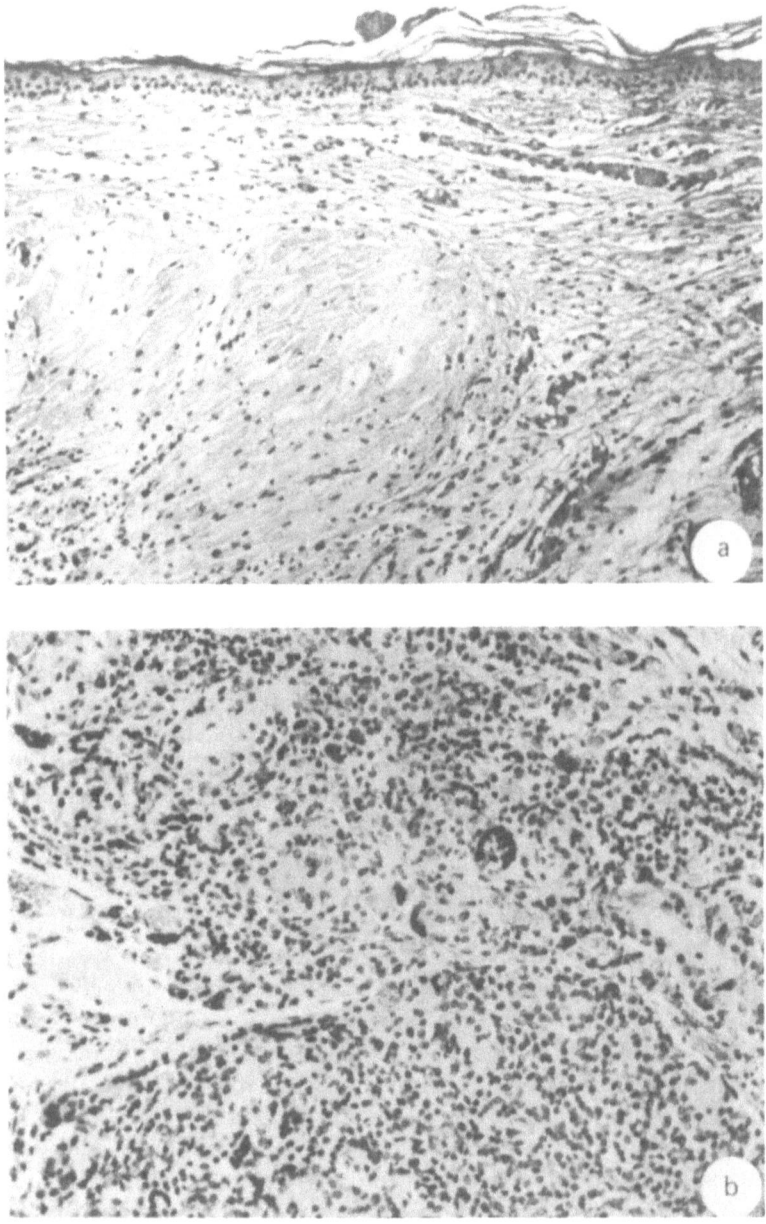

Fig. 42 a–d.   Patterns of delayed rejection. **a.** Biopsy at zero end point of rapid, chronic, first-set allograft rejection. A well-outlined collagen pad of residual graft connective tissue is present in the middermis. **b.** Biopsy at 10 days after zero end point of rapid, chronic, first-set allograft rejection. A marked granulomatous reaction in the deep dermis is present.

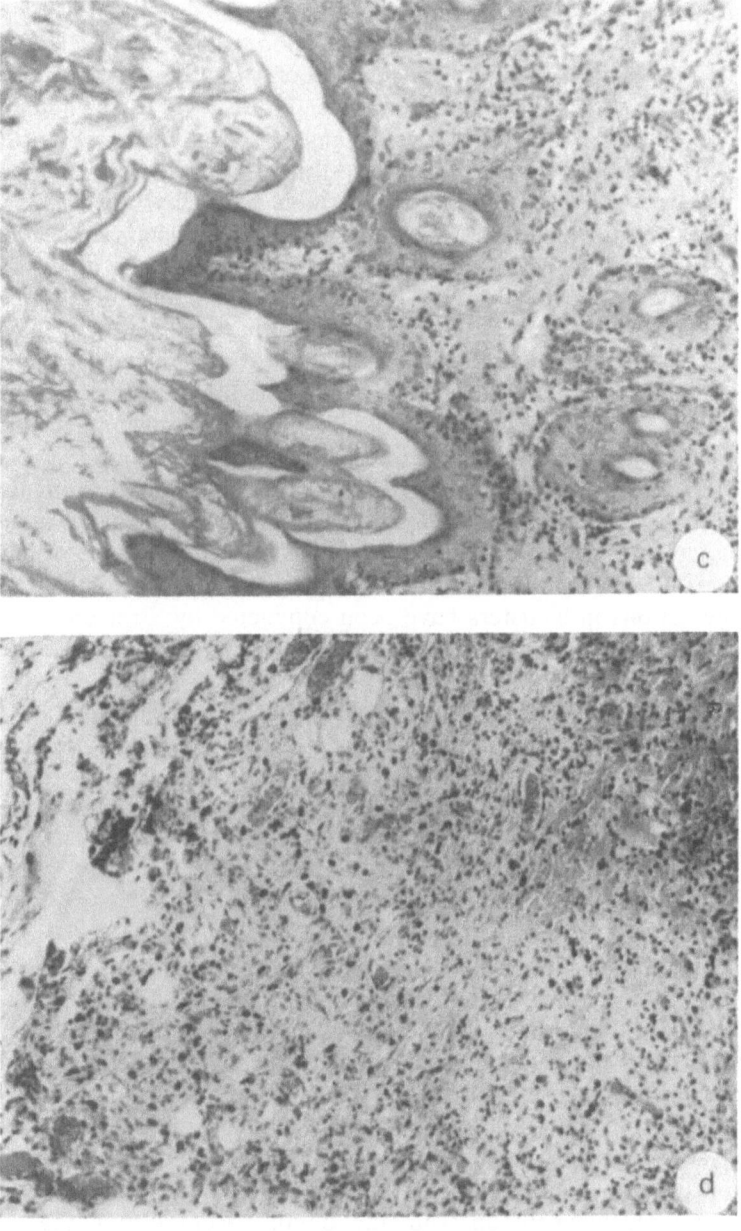

Fig. 42 *(Continued)* **c.** Early phase of prolonged chronic allograft rejection. The epidermis is greatly thickened and covered by a hyperkeratotic scale. **d.** Middle phase of prolonged chronic allograft rejection. Large numbers of mast cells *(intensely dark cells)* are scattered throughout the dermis. Hildemann and Walford (1960) Ann. N.Y. Acad. Sci. 87:56.

The findings of Billingham and Hildemann (1958a, b) showing prompt rejection of skin allografts in certain donor–host strain combinations suggested the possibility of the existence of only one or two major histocompatibility loci (or genes) in these animals. To test this theory, Billingham, Sawchuck, and Silvers (1960) transplanted full-thickness skin allografts among the members of three disparate strains of Syrian hamsters and also from the parental and grandparental strains to F_2 hybrids. The grafting techniques and diagnostic criteria described by Billingham and Hildemann (1958b) were followed with slight modifications. From the analysis of the survival times of skin allografts between the members of various strain combinations and their F_2 progeny, Billingham et al. (1960) concluded that an acute reaction of allograft rejection in the Syrian hamster is governed by one or two histocompatibility genes responsible for transplantation immunity, whereas the high compatibility of skin grafts depends on a single minor histocompatibility gene associated with weak graft rejection.

Although histocompatibility genetics and transplantation immunology have not yet been as extensively studied in the Syrian hamster as in other species, preliminary experiments to demonstrate the presence of the major histocompatibility complex, graft-versus-host reactions, and mixed lymphocyte interactions in hamsters have been conducted by Streilein and Billingham (1970a, b), Singh and Tevethia (1973), and most recently by Duncan and Streilein (1978a, b).

Although the gross and histologic features of skin allografts in the hamster during the course of chronic rejection have been described in detail by all of the investigators cited, there has been no reference to the graft vascular pattern relative to the various phases of the immune reaction.

Family Studies

Inspired by the previous experience of Peer (1956), who observed the prolonged survival of an experimental skin graft from a mother to her infant who had been given maternal blood intramuscularly when newly born, Peer, Bernhard, and Walker (1958) exchanged a series of full-thickness skin grafts from the posterior surface of the auricle between human parents and their children, mostly infants. They found that a number of the grafts between mother and son or daughter persisted for longer periods of time than those between the father–child pairs, regardless of whether or not the child received intramuscular blood from the donor parent during the neonatal period. They concluded that the tolerance, relative or complete, of the mother–child recipients to each other's skin was not the result of prior conditioning of the child with donor blood. The authors stated that degenerative changes appearing in some of the tolerated grafts were not always destructively progressive but seemed to be reversible. Some of these transplants recovered from the initial circulatory embarrassment and proceeded to heal in a normal fashion; nevertheless they were eventually rejected at a later date and replaced by host tissue.

Rogers, Raisbeck, Ballantyne, and Converse (1960) reported similar results in closely related rats. In some grafts, early signs of disturbance in blood flow and in the character of graft vessels, which might otherwise have progressively led to complete cessation of blood flow and eventual vascular disruption, suddenly disappeared without further evidence that the graft was being rejected. Such a graft was then rejected at a later period by gradual elimination in a matter of many weeks or months, usually with the formation of a linear scar. With regard to this particular type of chronic rejection, it should be noted that under a variety of controlled experimental conditions, several earlier investigators, such as Anderson, Billingham, Lampkin, and Medawar (1951), Billingham, Krohn, and Medawar (1951), Billingham and Medawar (1951), and Dammin and Murray (1959), mentioned the formation of a scar after a drawn out latent period.

Further evidence of prolonged graft survival was obtained by Peer in 1957 and again in 1958 from human patients. In these studies reciprocal skin grafts were transferred between parents and their young offspring. It was concluded that mothers are superior to fathers as skin donors to their children. Allografts from mothers survived considerably longer than those from fathers, up to 250 days. However, the status of the blood supply in the grafts when they were undergoing the rejection reaction was not described.

It was reported by Rogers (1957a) that skin grafts taken from closely related human donors transplanted to healthy recipients under strict control conditions survive longer than those from unrelated donors. The sequence of vascular events in the grafts with prolonged survival was not described; there was only a cursory reference to thromboses, hemorrhages, and extravasation into the graft dermis.

Results obtained from family studies in humans have elicited considerable attention because skin grafts removed from a closely related donor can survive for prolonged periods when used to resurface areas of skin destroyed by burns. Furthermore, questions have been posed as to whether further differences exist among grafts interchanged between members of the same family, as well as between relatives of different age categories. To explore this possibility Rogers et al. (1960), working with closely related but not inbred rats, initiated an intensive investigation on the average survival time of skin transplanted from parents and other closely related donors, such as siblings and grandparents, to the untreated infants. The techniques of gross and stereomicroscopic observations of graft behavior developed by Taylor and Lehrfeld (1953) was adopted for this experiment.

The findings at periodic time intervals substantiated the human studies of Peer (1958) and showed that all grafts exchanged between the father and his offspring, either male or female, were rapidly rejected in the usual fashion. Longer survival occurred in grafts from the offspring to the father; the longest survival time being 39 days. In contrast to this, a significant percentage, approximately 25%, of the grafts exchanged between a mother and her offspring underwent prolonged survival; some grafts were still viable at 204 days. At this time the rat recipients were sacrificed for histologic assay.

Of particular note is the report by Ceppellini *et al.* (1966), who studied skin grafts in healthy human subjects under a stereomicroscope (see page 65). In vivo observations of full-thickness orthotopic skin grafts showed that ABO-compatible grafts reciprocally transplanted between siblings tended to survive significantly longer than those between unrelated individuals. However, there was no significant difference in survival time between father-to-child and mother-to-child allografts, in contradiction to the previous findings of Peer (1958).

In 1978, further claims of improvement in the survival times of ABO-compatible skin allografts exchanged between members of 97 white families were made by Ward, Mendell, Seigler, MacQueen, and Amos. It was determined that skin allografts derived from HLA-identical siblings tend to survive significantly longer than those from siblings, parents, or others clearly mismatched for one or two haplotypes. Consistent with this conclusion are the findings that the longest survival time recorded for grafts between HLA-identical siblings is 24.9 ± 0.9 days, in contrast to that of 14.8 ± 0.3 days for haploidentical grafts and 12.1 ± 0.7 days for grafts between siblings differing at both haplotypes. In this regard, it is also apparent that haploidentical grafts survive significantly longer than those between siblings who differ at two haplotypes. Another interesting aspect of this clinical study is that the sex of the donor and recipient has no demonstrable influence on the survival of haploidentical grafts (15.0 ± 0.6 days for grafts from male or female to female versus 14.7 ± 0.7 days for grafts from female or male to male).

Other lines of clinical evidence indicate that among the HLA-identical and haploidentical family members significant improvement in survival of grafts ($p < 0.01$) is seen in older recipients. From the comparative evaluation of skin allografts between haploidentical individuals, it is apparent that grafts with one mismatched antigen survive longer than those with two mismatched antigens. This difference (1.4 days), as cited by the authors, is only one-half of that between one and no mismatched antigens (2.9 days). It was also reported that the location of the mismatched antigens at the A locus or B locus of the HLA system has no apparent effect on the graft survival.

Rogers *et al.* (1960) stressed, as did Hildemann and Walford (1960) in the Syrian hamster, that the survival end points of skin allografts transplanted between closely related but not inbred rats are not always clear-cut or distinct. Under direct skin stereomicroscopy, complete hemal stasis or vascular disruption, which is usually seen after 1 week, or shortly thereafter, in graft interchanges between unrelated rats, is observed between related members only if the grafts are undergoing a typical rapid or acute rejection. Other grafts, however, undergo a slower or chronic rejection, which Rogers

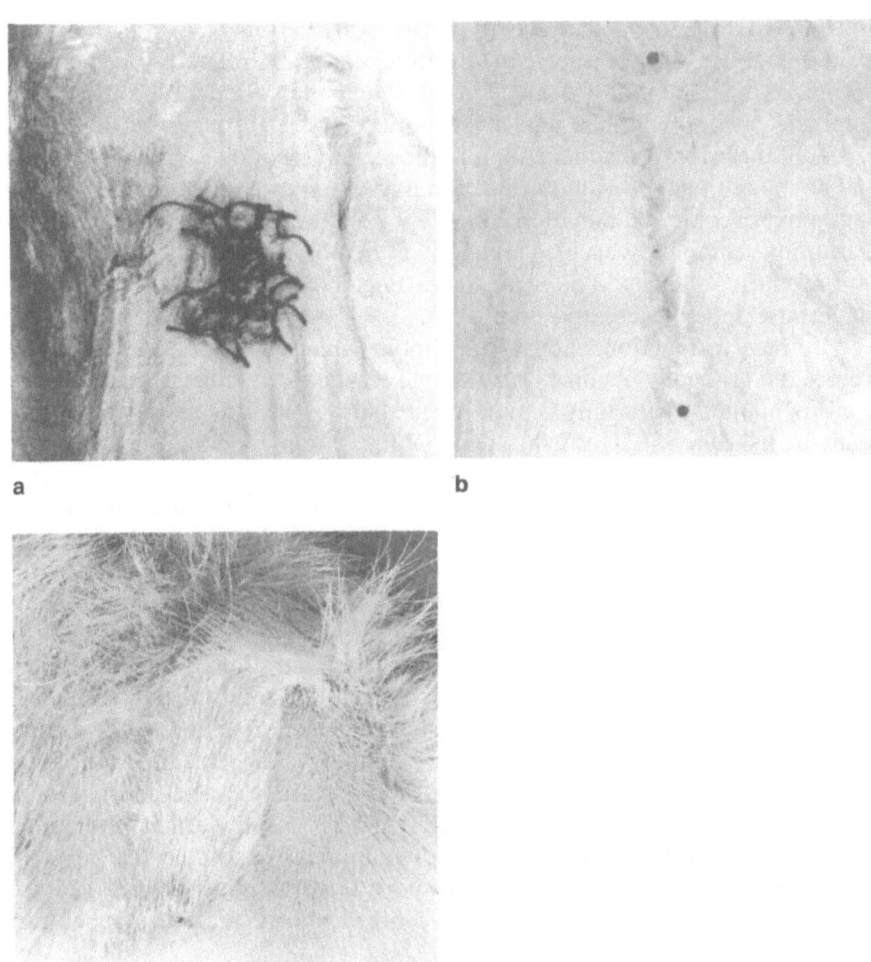

Fig. 43 a–c. Examples of scab and scar reactions of chronic rejection and prolonged survival in grafts between related rats. **a.** Scab reaction which appeared suddenly 43 days after a brother's skin allograft was transplanted to his sister. Sutures had been purposefully left in place to demarcate the edge of the graft. **b.** Scar reaction *(between black dots)* 57 days after transplantation. The allograft has gradually shrunk from its original margins to a fine, linear hairless scar, but without evidence of hemal stasis or vascular breakdown in the slowly shrinking graft itself. **c.** Excellent appearance of a graft still present after 202 days, at which time the animal was sacrificed for histologic study. Rogers, Raisbeck, Ballantyne, and Converse (1960) Transactions of the International Society of Plastic Surgeons, Second Congress, London. E. & S. Livingstone, Edinburgh, p. 421.

and his associates (1960) have termed the *scab* (Fig. 43a) and the *scar reactions* (Fig. 43b). In the scab reaction, the graft frequently appears as normal as an autograft for many weeks, and then suddenly undergoes a complete change within a day or so until a dry scab occupies the entire extent of the graft. A few hours before the formation of the scab, the survival end points of this type of graft rejection have been categorized under in vivo stereomicroscopic examination either by complete hemal stasis, vascular disruption, complete vascular breakdown, hemorrhagic loci, or a combination of these changes. The scab, in essence, represents loss of the graft epidermis, appendages, and dermis.

In the scar reaction, the graft resembles an autograft for many days or weeks, but gradually becomes smaller and smaller, seeming to shrink slowly from its margins, with only a thin, linear, hairless scar as the eventual end point of its survival. Until this end point is attained, however, vascular changes and the rate of blood circulation appear normal under stereomicroscopic inspection, and, since all grafts are intentionally rotated when transplanted in order to facilitate identification, the reversed growth of its hair pattern continues to be evident.

According to Ballantyne (1960), from histologic observation of representative skin biopsies taken from some rats in the preceding study, the scar reaction is characterized by a mild lymphocytic infiltration occurring primarily at the dermoepidermal junction of the graft and the demarcation line between the graft and host. This invasive lymphocytic response is accompanied by a perivascular infiltration of lymphocytes, specifically around the graft vessels. In addition, the dermis of the graft remnant consists of a narrow upper dermal layer and an increasingly wider dermal layer as it proceeds downward to the graft base. The findings suggested that most of the original graft epidermis and upper portion of the graft dermal pad are absorbed and replaced by the host at a more rapid rate than the deeper part of the dermal pad.

In prolonged survival, most of the allografts are still viable at 204 days, as manifested by the reversed growth of the hair crop (Fig. 43c). At this stage, the surviving graft is microscopically identifiable only by a slight thickening of the graft collagen fibers, particularly at the union line between the graft and host, coupled with a diffuse and mild lymphocytic infiltration in the graft dermis.

Summary

There are several convincing lines of evidence in the published reports that skin allografts between genetically dissimilar individuals, instead of undergoing a typical rapid or acute rejection, may enjoy longer periods of survival in healthy recipients without any chemotherapeutic or immunosuppressive treatment. Variations of a delayed immunologic response of rejection by the host and protracted graft survival have been observed in certain animal species, mostly the Syrian hamster, and specific familial donor–host combinations, especially mother-to-child grafts, in closely related human individuals and rats. A variety of diagnostic assay techniques, particularly visual inspection and touch-palpation, direct skin stereomicroscopy, and histology, have been employed to assess the sequence of events in the grafts with prolonged survival.

If an allograft is not rejected acutely or violently, it may undergo a slower or chronic reaction that ranges, in order of increasing survival times, from a rapid chronic reaction with a slightly prolonged graft survival, through a slower chronic reaction with a slightly longer survival, to very prolonged graft survival. Despite the type of chronic reactions or the length of graft survival times, all allografts (including those that undergo acute rejection) are initially nourished by serum imbibition and subsequently by the restoration of an adequate blood supply from the host during the first few days after transplantation. However, after complete vascularization of the graft, the sequence of events in the chronic reaction (in which the length of the survival time varies), unlike that observed in the acute rejection reaction, consists of (1) a delayed mild to moderate inflammatory response, (2) slower rates of breakdown and replacement of different tissue components in the graft by host cells, and (3) longer latent periods and delayed onset of the immunologic response of graft rejection.

Chapter 4

Reaction Patterns of Skin Xenografts

Biologic Behavior

The mode of vascularization and the course of tissue morphology and vascular changes following the transplantation of skin xenografts have not been extensively investigated. It has been generally held that skin transplanted between members of different species induces a more rapid and violent rejection reaction than do allografts. According to Ribbert-Göttingen (1904), who transplanted skin from humans and guinea pigs to rabbits, xenografts were rejected within 3 days after transplantation. Loeb and Addison (1909, 1911) reported that skin xenografts interchanged between various animals, including rats, mice, guinea pigs, rabbits, cats, and even pigeons, eventually became necrotic after 6–11 days and occasionally even more rapidly. They did not provide information regarding either the vascularization or the vascular pattern of the xenografts. Woodruff (1960) maintained that xenografts show little or no evidence of vascularization and that ischemia rather than rejection is responsible for the lack of success of the xenografts. Indeed, for a long time most authorities agreed that xenografts invariably fail to receive a direct blood supply from the recipient before the onward rush of the rejection phenomenon.

However, during the past two decades there have been indications in the literature that skin xenografts, particularly among certain rodents, are capable of being revascularized from the host bed. There have also been reports of the distention of blood vessels, breakdown of the endothelial wall, clotting of blood, and focal hemorrhages in the dermis of a skin xenograft undergoing rejection; these reactions are identical to those described in allograft breakdown.

Studies with the Chick Embryo as a Graft Recipient

Early Phases of Graft Survival

It was originally reported by Murphy (1912, 1913, 1914a) that various malignant tumors and embryonic cells taken from the rat, mouse, and human could be successfully transplanted to the developing chick embryo. However, Kiyono and Sueyasu (1917) appear to be the first to report the transplantation of normal organized tissues, including skin, on the chorioallantoic membrane of the chick embryo and to describe the absorption of nutrient fluids by the graft from the embryonic tissue and the actual entry of avian blood vessels into the graft. Goodpasture, Douglas, and Anderson (1938) reported the revascularization and growth of split-thickness human skin grafts transplanted to the chorioallantois of the chick embryo; the presence of nucleated chick red blood cells in the graft was considered presumptive evidence of vascular ingrowth, an observation originally described by Murphy (1912). The chorionic capillaries penetrate the undersurface of the human skin dermis within 48 hours after grafting, and by 3 or 4 days the network of endothelial channels in the graft contains avian nucleated erythrocytes. Goodpasture et al. (1938) accepted the concept of the direct connection of host and graft vessels because their histologic sections demonstrated a mixture of human and chick red blood cells. However, they implied that while there is ample evidence favoring anastomoses between the vasculature of the human skin transplant and that of the avian membrane as well as capillary ingrowth from the host into the undersurface of the graft, they do not permit active blood flow in the graft. The nourishment of the graft is primarily derived through the temporary vascular communication between the two vascular systems.

In the section on Phase of Serum Imbibition in Chapter 1, there was a brief review of a report by Converse and associates (1957) describing the early nourishment of rabbit skin xenografts by rapid fluid uptake from the chorioallantoic membrane of the chick embryo during the first 24 hours.

Further attempts to define the mode of vascularization of skin xenografts from man and various animal species transplanted to the surface of the chorioallantoic membrane of an embryo were undertaken by Converse, Ballantyne, Rogers, and Raisbeck (1958), who adopted the modified chick chorioallantois method of Goodpasture et al. (1938). Differences in structure between the mammalian erythrocytes and the nucleated avian erythrocytes (Fig. 44a) made it possible to determine that the definitive vasculature of the full-thickness skin xenografts of rabbit, rat, and bovine embryo is provided mainly by the host vascular ingrowth into the graft (Fig. 44b) while the original vessels of the grafts degenerate. When human skin of varying thickness is applied to the chorioallantois of the chick, the major definitive vasculature capable of supporting an active circulation between graft and

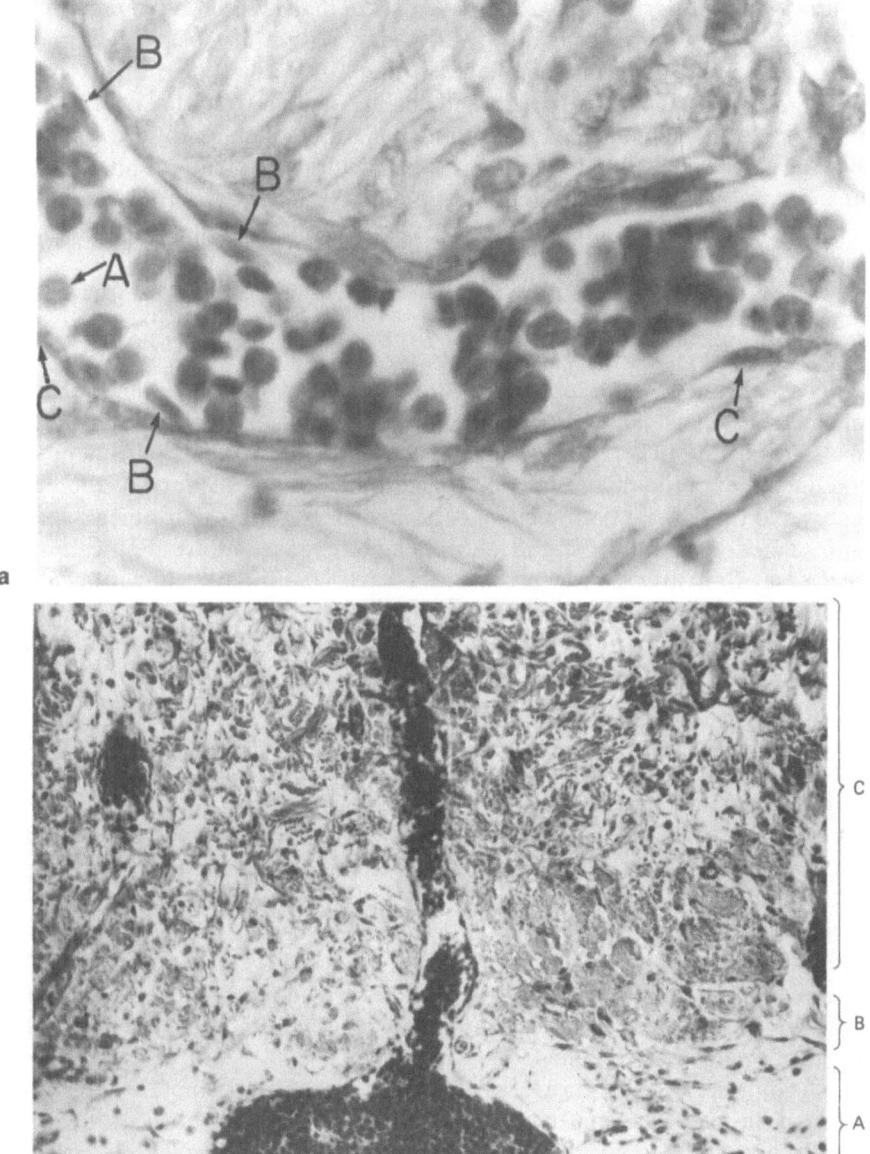

Fig. 44 a and b. Revascularization of xenografts implanted in chick embryo. **a.** A membranal blood vessel in the human dermis contains both human *(A)* and chick *(B)* erythrocytes 4 days after grafting. Note the clear outline of the endothelial lining *(C)*. ×440. **b.** Note the deep penetration of an embryonal blood vessel from the chorioallantois *(A)* through the union line *(B)* into the dermis *(C)* of the freeze-dried bovine skin graft 5 days after grafting. ×102. Converse, Ballantyne, Rogers, and Raisbeck (1958) Transplant. Bull. 5:108, © (1958) The Williams & Wilkins Co., Baltimore.

host is similarly derived from the progressive ingrowth of avian endothelial cells into the graft. There is also rapid deterioration of most of the original graft vessels. In addition, histologic studies by Ballantyne and Converse (1958) of composite grafts of skin and cartilage taken from the auricle of the rabbit and transplanted to the chorionic membrane of chick embryos showed that the embryonal blood vessels make a tortuous course around the cartilage barrier (Fig. 45) and eventually penetrate into the dermis above the cartilage. Meanwhile, most of the preexisting vessels in the auricular grafts degenerate.

Rejection Mechanism in the Chick Embryo

It is recognized that the chick embryo is capable of developing defensive mechanisms that result in the rejection of normal tissue and tumor transplants (Murphy 1914a, b; Green and Lorincz 1956). There is limited but convincing experimental evidence that the immune resistance of the chick embryo to foreign skin often appears immediately prior to, or coincidentally with, the degeneration of the chorioallantoic vasculature. For example, Converse, Ballantyne, Rogers, and Raisbeck (1958) have shown that incipient signs of a necrotic process appear in the dermis of a few skin grafts 7 days after transplantation, or on the 17th day of embryonic development. An increasing number of grafts show partial or complete necrosis of the dermis by day 8 following transplantation, which is the 18th day of incubation. On day 10 after grafting, the last day of the incubation period, most of the grafts show a degenerative appearance, an intense proliferation of leukocytes of various types, and keratinization of the epidermis. However, there are some instances in which the degenerative changes in the graft do not occur, and in other situations deterioration of the chorioallantoic membrane, chorioallantoic vasculature, and graft occur concurrently. Histologic findings appear to corroborate the gross observations of a yellow color, slight shrinkage in circumference, and thickening of the graft, usually on day 8 or 9 after transplantation. It should also be noted that, whether or not the grafts are rejected by the end of the embryonic development, they are invariably damaged or lost at hatching.

Additional data that suggest that immune mechanisms are developed prior to the degeneration of the chorioallantoic vasculature were obtained from experiments in which human skin grafts were retransplanted from one embryo to another. Goodpasture et al. (1938) were usually unsuccessful in attempts to retransplant the grafts from one embryo at 8 days for the first transfer, and at 6 days for the second transfer. Blank, Coriell, and Scott (1948) successfully made serial retransplants of human skin grafts at 7-day intervals, keeping them alive for 27 days. It would appear that the capacity to reject the transplant occurs 7–8 days after transplantation, or on the 17th or 18th day of embryonic development.

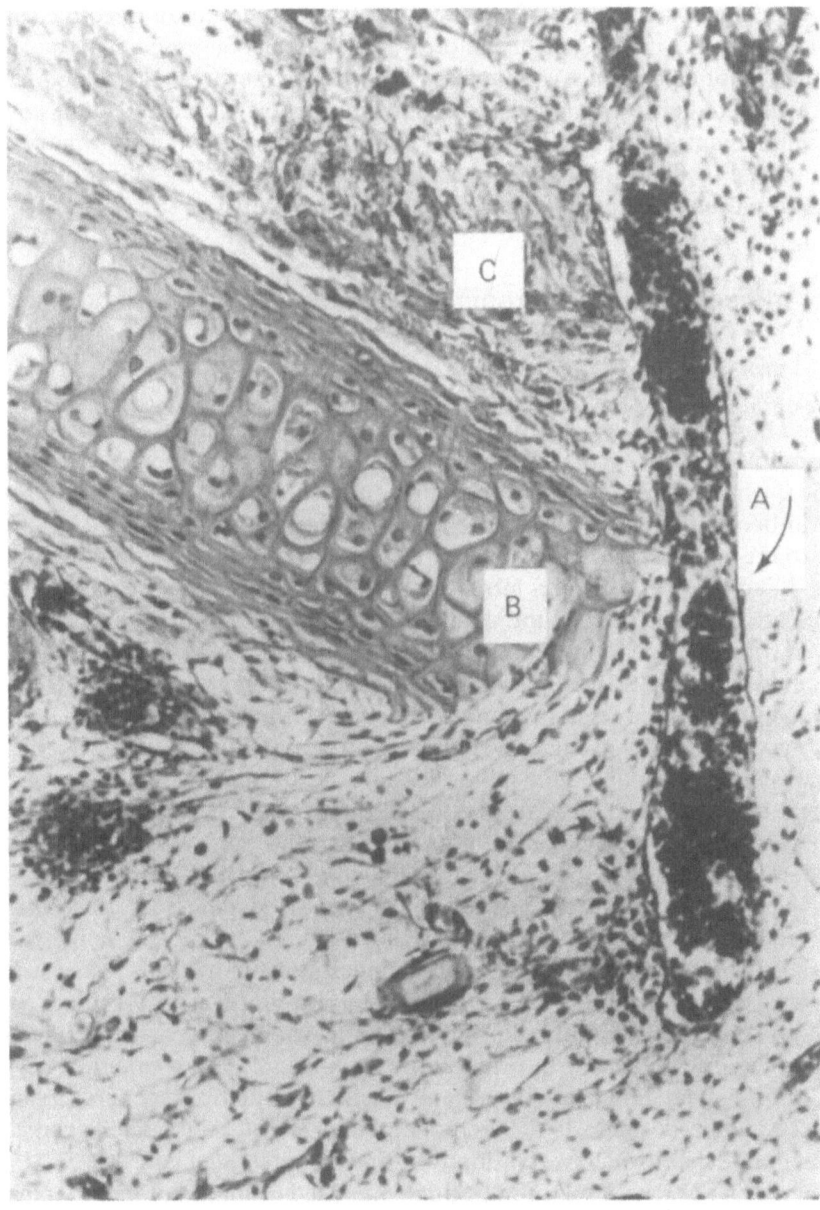

Fig. 45. Composite skin and cartilage graft from rabbit auricle transplanted to chorionic membrane of chick embryo. Note the migration of the chick blood vessel *(A)* around the end of the cartilage *(B)* penetrating into the dermis *(C)* of the composite graft. ×112. Ballantyne and Converse (1958) Transplant. Bull. 5:373, © (1958) The Williams & Wilkins Co., Baltimore.

Because the capacity of the chick embryo to mount an effective resistance against normal tissue or tumor transplants becomes evident at or close to the end of embryonic development, very few experimental attempts have been undertaken to examine the manifestations of tissue rejection in the recipient embryo. This lack of data is in sharp contrast to the information on the source of fluid nourishment and blood supply in grafts placed over the embryonal membrane of chicks.

Experiments with Orthotopic Xenografts

Stereomicroscopic Observations

Blood flow was observed in the vasculature of skin xenografts removed from the rabbit or mouse and transferred to a recipient rat by Egdahl *et al.* (1957, 1958), whereas transplants from the rat, mouse, or guinea pig to the rabbit never became effectively vascularized nor adhered to the host bed. According to the authors, who used the in vivo stereomicroscopic method of Taylor and Lehrfeld (1953) and an intradermal fluorescein test as their criteria for circulation (see page 23), the donor skin of the mouse or rabbit placed on the rat recipients is vascularized more slowly and has a shorter period of circulatory function than is usually seen in skin allografts. Blood flow in the xenografts is usually initiated on the fourth or fifth day after grafting, attains the maximal rate of circulation soon thereafter, continues at this velocity for only a few hours, and suddenly ceases on or around the sixth day. It has been suggested that the vasculature of the xenografts capable of bearing blood flow is not newly formed, but represents the original graft vasculature system, which establishes a direct connection with that of the host.

The incipient signs of rejection in a vascularized xenograft as seen under a stereomicroscope are the slowing of the blood flow, complete hemal stasis, vascular thrombosis, and small multiple necrotic hemorrhages. The average survival times for rabbit-to-rat and mouse-to-rat grafts are 5.9 and 6.1 days, respectively, considerably shorter than that of allografts in rats, which is 10.1 days. Intradermally injected fluorescein usually fades in either normal or grafted skin, showing an adequate vascular circulation; its persistence in these xenografts supports the stereomicroscopic criteria for the diagnosis of rejection. Histologic observations of Egdahl and associates (1957, 1958) indicate an intense cellular infiltration composed primarily of mature plasma cells, with moderate amounts of lymphocytes and macrophages, in the graft bed prior to the onset of overt tissue rejection. A parallel finding is the perivascular infiltration of all blood vessels in the graft and the formation of a wide cuff of lymphocytes and plasma cells. The findings of leukocytic infiltration in the graft bed and around the vessels and vascular damage in vascularized xenografts suggest a form of inflammatory reaction similar in some ways to the Arthus reaction.

Rolle *et al.* (1959) exchanged full-thickness skin grafts between mice and rats and found that the early sequence of vascular events occurring in the xenografts is similar to that in autografts and allografts (see page 24). As shown by stereomicroscopy, histology, and the injection of dyes, the onset and restoration of circulation as well as other vascular changes in xenografts prior to the rejection reaction are similar to those seen in allografts of mice or rats. The authors contended that the blood supply in the xenografts is restored by the establishment of continuity between the host and graft vessels.

The gross, stereomicroscopic, and histologic manifestations of resistance to skin xenografts resemble those seen in allografts of mouse or rat skin (see the section on Assessment of Graft Behavior by a Combination of Various Assay Methods in Chapter 2), with the exception of the survival time; the survival time of xenografts is shorter by 1 or 2 days. The authors concluded that the events that characterize the rejection of xenografts, similar to those of the Arthus reaction, are the direct result of vascular failure.

In 1969 Ballantyne, Uhlschmid, and Converse transplanted full-thickness skin grafts from the flanks and auricles of rabbits to suprapannicular skin defects on the dorsum of rats. Based on daily gross and stereomicroscopic observations, they confirmed the findings of Egdahl *et al.* (1958), showing strong tissue adhesion between the graft and host and the reestablishment of a major definitive vasculature, in which brisk blood flow occurred in most grafts by 3–4 days after transplantation. However, unlike most autografts and allografts, which normally assume a pinkish hue shortly after grafting, all xenografts appeared consistently pale, even with strong stereomicroscopic evidence of a rapid blood flow in the graft vessels. In addition, a small degree of edema, characteristically seen in the xenografts on the first day after transplantation, had subsided by the third or fourth day.

The earliest indication of the onset of rejection is the increased distention of graft vessels, followed rapidly by complete cessation of blood flow, vascular disruption, and tissue hardening, usually between the sixth and eighth day after grafting. The grafts also exhibit glossy transparence in the dermal tissue between the disrupted tissue and rapidly become opaque, characterized by complete coalescence of discolored areas over the entire graft surface.

Considerable attention was given by Ben-Hur *et al.* (1969a) to the response of mice to circular xenografts of full-thickness skin removed from rabbits, guinea pigs, and rats. Daily gross and direct skin stereomicroscopic examinations after the method of Taylor and Lehrfeld (1953) were performed to diagnose the status of blood flow and the physical condition of the grafts. The findings were correlated with serial histologic studies.

The response of mice to rat skin xenografts was characterized by early mononuclear and polymorphonuclear infiltration of the grafts, varying degrees of vascularization and blood circulation, and rapid epithelial degenera-

tion of the graft epidermis and its appendages. Grafts that had been successfully vascularized by the third day following transplantation showed an
abrupt cessation of blood flow, thrombosis, and hemorrhage on the third and
fourth day; other grafts that had failed to be vascularized showed the typical
features of the avascular white graft reaction (see the section on the White
Graft Reaction in Chapter 7), progressing into tan-colored eschars by the
fifth to seventh day. The remainder of the grafts underwent a course of
mixed white graft rejection, which, by gross stereomicroscopic and histologic criteria, is neither a typical accelerated reaction nor a typical white
graft reaction.

    In contrast to the rat grafts, most of the guinea pig grafts applied to
mouse recipients were characterized by an absence of vascularization.
There were a few instances, however, of an abortive attempt at vascular
penetration into the graft base and a particularly prominent infiltration of
mononuclear and fibroblastlike cells at the graft base (Fig. 46a). Such grafts

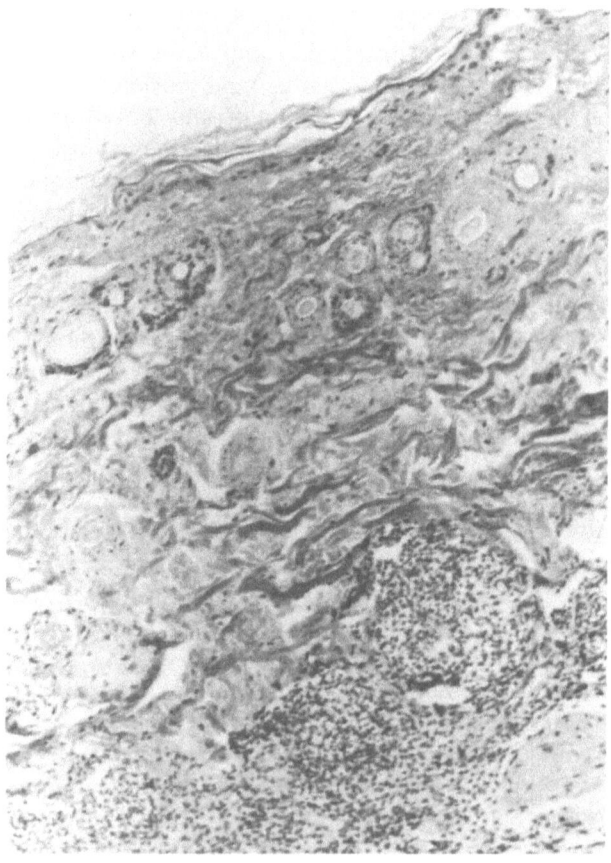

Fig. 46a. *Legend on facing page.*

underwent either one of two courses of the rejection process: most grafts underwent a typical white graft reaction, while others underwent a mixed white graft reaction.

Stereomicroscopic observations of the rabbit grafts on the mouse showed no evidence of graft vascularization or circulating blood for the first 3 days after grafting. At 4 days multiple vessels were filled with blood (Fig.

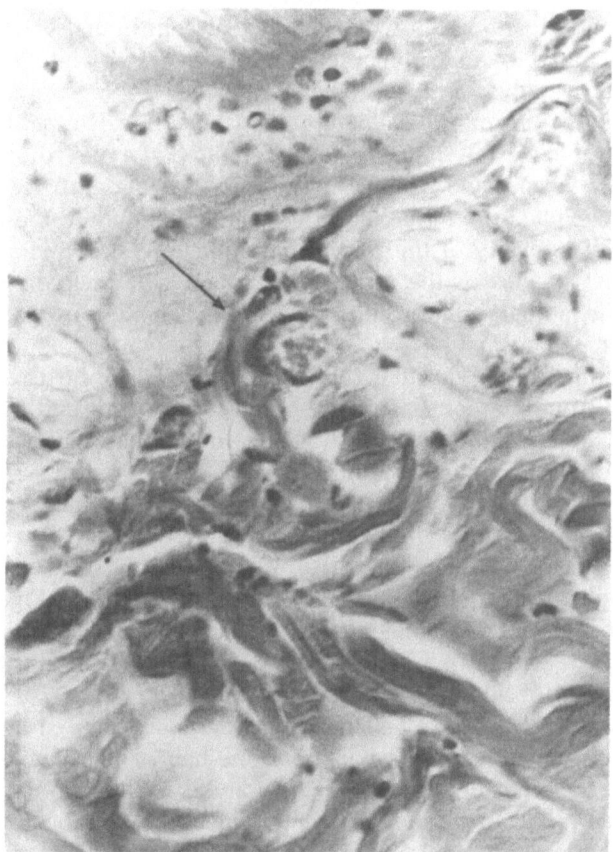

Fig. 46b

Fig. 46 a and b. Failure of guinea pig and rabbit xenografts transplanted to mice to revascularize. **a.** Guinea pig to mouse xenograft 4 days after transplantation. Note the epidermal thinning and necrosis, degeneration of epidermal appendages, disorganization of dermis, prominent mixed cell infiltrate, and congestion of vessels at the base of the graft. H & E. ×75. **b.** Rabbit to mouse xenograft 4 days after transplantation. Note the degeneration of the epidermis and epidermal elements and the disorganization of the dermis. Multiple small vessels filled with blood are present in the graft. H & E. ×325. Ben-Hur, Solowey, and Rapaport (1969) Isr. J. Med. Sci. 5:1.

46b) but did not manifest circulation; occasional thrombi and punctuate hemorrhages could be seen. In contrast to this observation, on histologic examination, numerous vessels filled with blood were found at all levels of the graft dermis at 3 days. As pointed out by the authors, there is no clear association between stereomicroscopic and histologic findings in regard to graft vascularization. Shortly thereafter, the rabbit xenografts exhibited vascular disruption, hemorrhages, necrosis and lysis of the epidermis, and prominent participation of polymorphonuclear cells in the rejection process. Such degenerative changes, characteristic of a mixed white graft rejection reaction, are usually completed by day 5.

Despite the information gained in this study, Ben-Hur et al. (1969a) did not provide a clear-cut interpretation for several types of xenograft responses, i.e., accelerated white graft and mixed white graft reactions. They also did not explain the mode of graft vascularization and the variations in the degree of intensity of the rejection response to skin xenografts from a single animal species or the variation between species. No reference was made to the actual relationship between the graft vascularity and immunologic mechanisms.

The nature of the vascular response of guinea pig hosts to skin xenografts taken from the mouse, rat, and rabbit was investigated by Ben-Hur et al. (1969b) in a subsequent work. They found that the reaction to the xenografts of all three species studied was basically a white graft (avascular) type of rejection (Fig. 47a), but some species showed a difference in the intensity of the reaction. Unlike auto- and allograft controls, the rat xenografts were not vascularized and there was no vascular penetration from the host during the first few days after transplantation (Fig. 47b). The xenogeneic response of guinea pigs to rat skin was invariably a pure white graft type of rejection in which the vascular breakdown and hemorrhagic necrosis typical of allograft rejection did not occur.

In contrast, the mouse and rabbit xenografts exhibited a mixed white graft type of rejection in approximately one-half of the histologic sections taken 4 and 5 days after surgery (Fig. 47c and d). When a mixed white graft reaction was involved, there was some evidence of an abortive attempt at revascularization, but without hemal flow, as manifested by occasional penetrating capillaries in the poor granulation tissue between graft and host. Blood cells were observed in some of these vessels. This may explain the occurrence of hemorrhages and capillary thromboses in some of the grafts that were undergoing a mixed white graft reaction.

Finally, in all species tested, the immune response was immediate, with a paucity of cellular infiltration during the early stages. According to Ben-Hur and his associates (1969b), the fact that guinea pigs actively rejected xenografts despite poor cellular reaction suggests a serologic response during the early stages, attributable to heterophile and other nonspecific antibodies.

Other Experimental Studies

The histologic and angiographic studies of Eastwood (1961) provided evidence that xenografts of pigskin applied to recipient rats are firmly adherent to the host bed, are successfully vascularized, and provide an effective cover for skin wound defects in the rat for an average of 10 days. The grafts appear grossly unchanged for the same duration of time before becoming dry and hard.

Bromberg, Song, and Mohn (1965), as did Song, Bromberg, Mohn, and Koehnlein (1966) in a subsequent experiment, injected 5% Evans blue into the femoral veins of recipient mice after porcine split-thickness skin xenografts had been applied to defects of the lower extremity. Following sacrifice of the animals, histologic study failed to show any evidence of revascularization in the xenografts or an immunologic inflammatory response of the host. In contrast, murine skin autografts and allografts demonstrated effective vascularization, even by the third day.

After transplanting porcine split-thickness skin grafts to mice, Pandya and Zarem (1974), using the transparant mouse chamber technique, noted that the host blood vessels in the near vicinity of transplants appeared slightly distended by the second day, but there was no demonstrable evidence of graft vascularization within 15 days after surgery.

With microangiographic techniques, Toranto, Salyer, and Myers (1974) demonstrated vascularization and viability of fresh full-thickness porcine skin on rabbit recipient sites by the third day. Their observations also indicated apparent vascularization of fresh pigskin grafts on the rat by 4 days, but the authors did not define the actual process by which the grafts received their blood supply. On the other hand, in the human host they were unable to distinguish between xenograft vascularization and invasion at the graft–host interface by granulation tissue. At 14 days there was no evidence of vascularization or viability of any xenografts, a finding consistent with rejection. Consequently, the authors recommended that when porcine skin is used as a biologic dressing the xenograft should be removed to minimize the risk of host sensitization.

Ben-Hur (1974), in commenting on the preceding work, stressed the importance of distinguishing between a freshly excised xenograft and a lyophilized, or formalin-fixed, xenograft when reporting on graft vascularization, tissue viability, and antigenic stimulus in provoking sensitization in the host. He was of the opinion that while a fresh xenograft is capable of being revascularized and initiating host antibody reaction, a lyophilized xenograft is dead and incapable of becoming vascularized and of participating in the rejection reaction, but may serve as a biologic dressing. In addition, when a fresh xenograft is applied as a biologic cover, the rejection reaction begins very early, sometimes almost immediately, probably due to the nonspecific heterophile antibodies. Consequently, there is a sluggishness

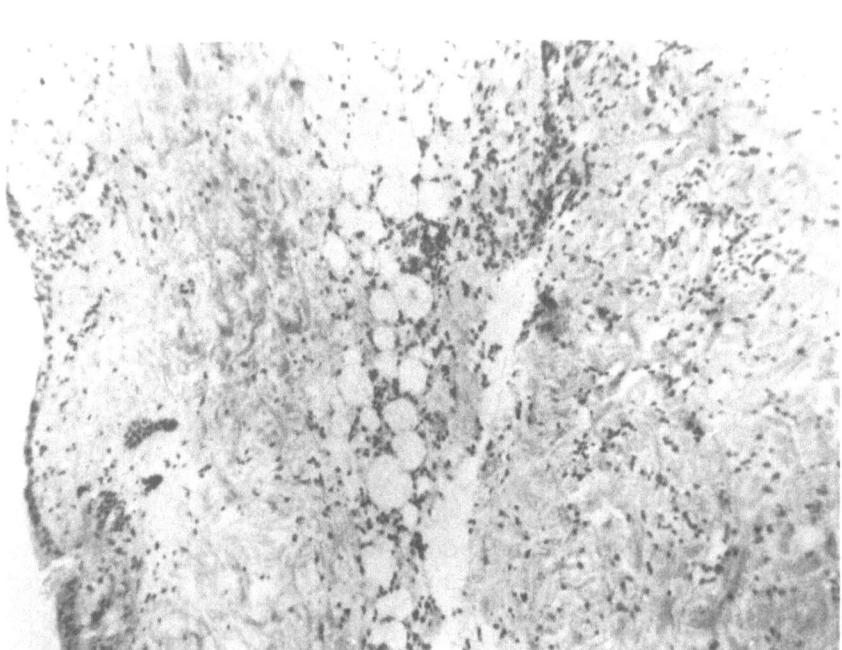

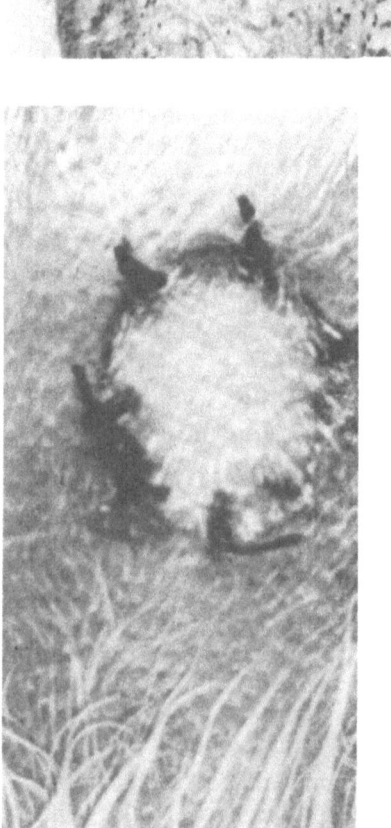

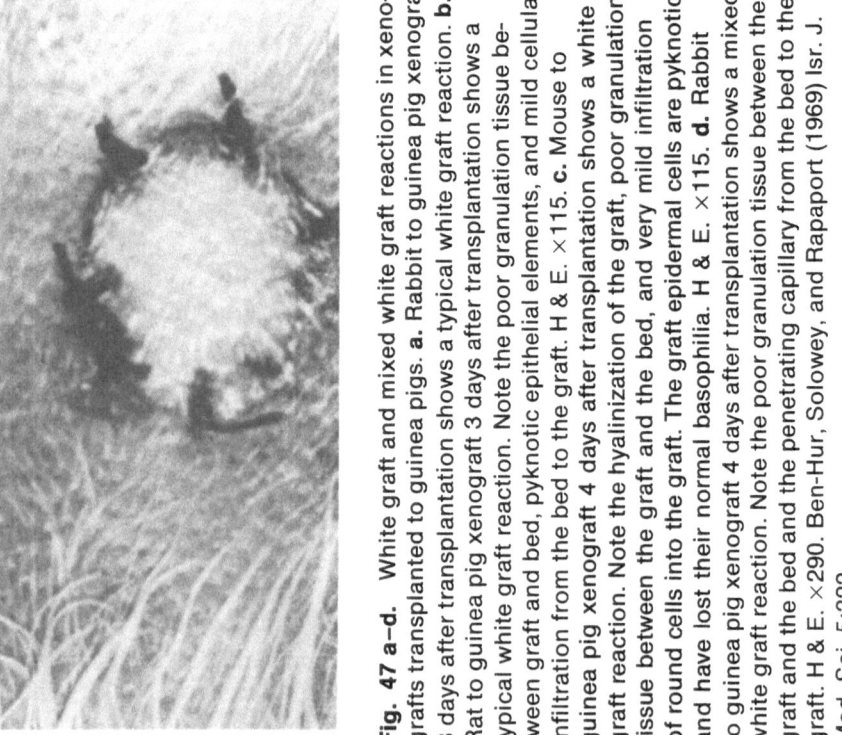

Fig. 47 a–d. White graft and mixed white graft reactions in xenografts transplanted to guinea pigs. **a.** Rabbit to guinea pig xenograft 3 days after transplantation shows a typical white graft reaction. **b.** Rat to guinea pig xenograft 3 days after transplantation shows a typical white graft reaction. Note the poor granulation tissue between graft and bed, pyknotic epithelial elements, and mild cellular infiltration from the bed to the graft. H & E. ×115. **c.** Mouse to guinea pig xenograft 4 days after transplantation shows a white graft reaction. Note the hyalinization of the graft, poor granulation tissue between the graft and the bed, and very mild infiltration of round cells into the graft. The graft epidermal cells are pyknotic and have lost their normal basophilia. H & E. ×115. **d.** Rabbit to guinea pig xenograft 4 days after transplantation shows a mixed white graft reaction. Note the poor granulation tissue between the graft and the bed and the penetrating capillary from the bed to the graft. H & E. ×290. Ben-Hur, Solowey, and Rapaport (1969) Isr. J. Med. Sci. 5:322.

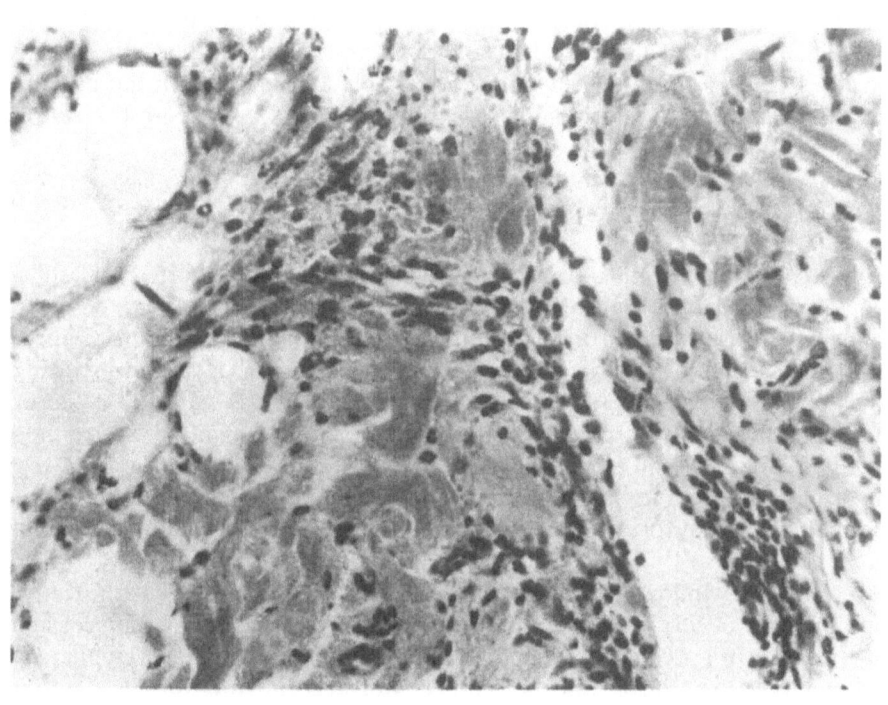

d

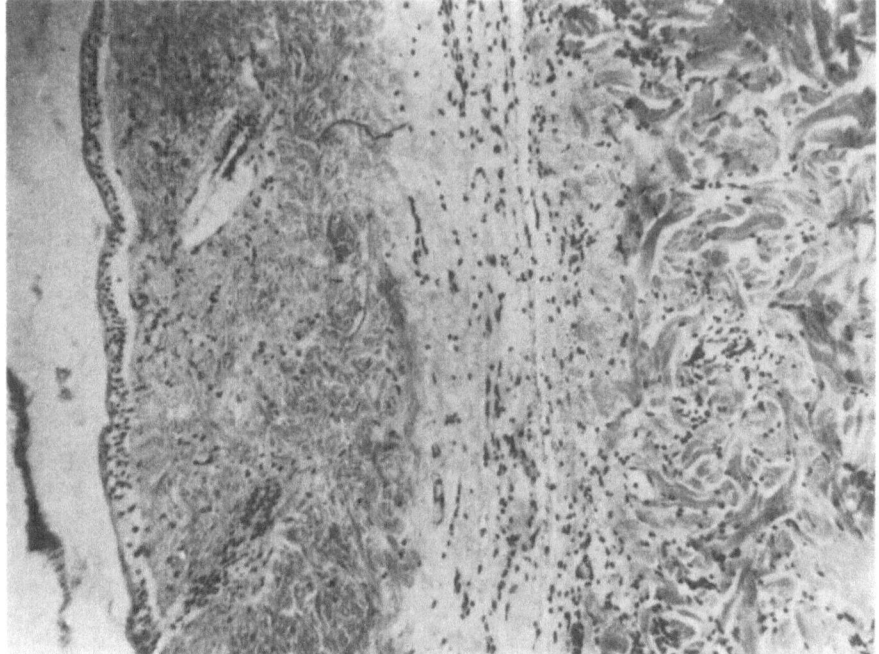

c

and stasis of the bed, accompanied by capillary breakdown in the graft, and petechiae appear. Thus, Ben-Hur attributes the failure of Toranto and associates (1974) to find any evidence of vessels and viability in the porcine skin xenografts by the 14th day after grafting to an early xenograft rejection response.

Studies on Skin Xenografts in Humans

Switzer, Moncrief, Mills, Order, and Lindberg, in 1966, reported that split-thickness skin grafts transplanted from 25 dogs to 30 patients proved to be satisfactory as biologic dressings in the management of thermal injury. Histologic examination of the tissue biopsies taken 4 days after grafting showed degenerating epidermis and intact dermis in the graft and a bed of immature but highly vascular granulation tissue containing many neutrophils and lymphocytes, and a few plasma cells. After 5 days the xenografts were so firmly adherent to the recipient sites that surgical removal was not possible, and therefore the rejection process had to be allowed to take its full course.

The skin window technique was employed by McCabe, Rebuck, Kelly, and Ditmars (1973) in human burn recipients who had received successive applications of porcine skin xenografts. An initial nonimmune, inflammatory cellular response during the first week after grafting was followed by an increasing immunocompetent cellular reaction that peaked at 30 days. Anti-pigskin humoral factors could not be detected. While there were no clinical manifestations of any host sensitization, such symptoms could have been masked by the usual stormy clinical course of severely burned patients.

Clinical Applications of Skin Xenografts

Rogers and Converse (1958) used experimental fetal calf skin xenografts as biologic dressings in humans and observed a surprising lack of host reaction to the fetal xenografts even after 12–17 days of graft retention. Bromberg *et al.* (1965) popularized the use of porcine xenografts as temporary biologic dressings. The function of skin xenografts as biologic dressings is similar to that outlined in the section on Indications for Skin Allografting in Man in Chapter 2.

Burleson and Eisman (1973) felt that the efficacy of biologic dressings could be attributed to their ability to adhere to tissue, and the adherence is due to a fibrin–elastin biologic bonding system. The same authors (1972) demonstrated that the unique adherent qualities of porcine skin were responsible for its antibacterial effect. They (1973) also questioned the role of neomycin and povidone-iodine solution (Betadine), used in the commercial preparation of porcine xenografts, and felt that these agents might be responsible for reducing surface bacterial counts.

While xenografts have been most extensively used in covering larger burn wounds prior to autografting, the use of xenografts has also been extended to the temporary coverage of exposed vessels, tendons, leg ulcers, flap donor sites, and skin graft donor sites (Elliott and Hoehn 1973; State and Peter 1974).

Salisbury, Wilmore, Silverstein, and Pruitt (1973) have cautioned against the application of porcine skin as temporary biologic dressings of skin graft donor sites because the incorporation of porcine collagen in the subepithelial area of the donor site may be detrimental. They found a significant incidence of donor site inflammation and delayed repair following the application of porcine xenografts.

Two cases of neomycin-induced nephrotoxicity and ototoxicity following the application of commercially prepared porcine skin xenografts have been reported. High neomycin blood levels were documented in both patients (Sugarbaker, Sabath, and Morgan 1974).

Summary

A variety of diagnostic assay methods have been employed for assessing the condition and status of orthotopic skin xenografts in their hosts. These methods have included visual inspection and touch-palpation of grafts in situ, stereomicroscopy in vivo, histologic examination of graft biopsy specimens, dye injections, and in vivo transplant chambers and microangiography. The experimental and clinical studies reviewed in this chapter produced astonishingly different results by different groups of investigators. Because there are conflicting reports, the controversy regarding graft vascularization and the course of tissue morphology and vascular events in xenografts is not yet settled. In addition, much discussion has arisen over whether xenografts are capable of stimulating a cellular inflammatory response, circulating humoral antibodies, and delayed hypersensitivity in the host similar to those observed in allografts. Of equal importance is the question of the involvement of graft vessels in provoking cellular and humoral responses in the recipient. Some authors have claimed that since skin xenografts are not vascularized, they do not cause local or systemic sensitivity in hosts.

Most investigators (Rogers, Converse, and Silvetti 1957; Rogers and Converse 1958; Song et al. 1966; Rappaport, Pepino, and Dietrick 1970; Silverstein, Munster, Curreri, and Pruitt 1971; State and Peter 1974) are of a similar opinion that skin xenografts do not elicit any significant cellular inflammatory response, humoral antibodies, or sensitization in the host. However, Sokolic, Farpour, Ulin, and Howard (1959), after transplanting fetal bovine skin grafts to dogs, noted strong polymorphonuclear infiltration at the graft–host junction, despite the lack of graft vascularization and transplantation immunity. Furthermore, McKhann and Berrian (1959a), using allografts, found, as did Etheredge, Shons, Harris, and Najarian (1971), using xenografts, that graft vascularization is not a prerequisite for the induction of transplantation immunity.

McCabe *et al.* (1973) stated that repeated applications of viable pigskin grafts to burned patients failed to provoke the production of circulating humoral antibodies in recipient sera. With a modification of the Terasaki leukocytic assay (1964), Harris and Abston (1974) demonstrated cytotoxic antibodies against pig lymphocytes in the sera of burned children but could not detect humoral antibody response to pigskin grafts. Law, Nathan, and MacMillan (1970), in an earlier study with animals and burned patients, also observed similar disparities between the lack of humoral antibody response to pigskin grafts and the successful development of cytotoxic responses to pig lymphocytes.

Other investigators (Egdahl *et al.* 1958; Rolle *et al.* 1959; Eastwood 1961; Ballantyne *et al.* 1969; Ben-Hur *et al.* 1969a, b; Toranto *et al.* 1974) showed that, depending on certain graft–host relationships and animal species combinations, particularly among rodents, skin xenografts become successfully vascularized, with stereomicroscopic evidence of active circulation and vascular distention. In addition, the extent, timing, and pattern of the immunologic response of the host to xenografts depend on the specific graft–host combination, varying from acute rejection similar to accelerated rejection of second-set allografts to mixed white and white graft reactions. The rejection of xenografts has been attributed by Egdahl and associates (1958) to the damage of the graft vessels by an inflammatory response similar to that which occurs in the Arthus reaction, and by Ben-Hur *et al.* (1968a, b) to the participation of polymorphonuclear leukocytes and nonspecific heterophile antibodies. In contrast, Toranto *et al.* (1974) suggested that interface contact between the host and graft could evoke host sensitization without the participation of graft vessels.

Chapter 5

Role of the Dosage Phenomenon in Allograft and Xenograft Reactions

Preliminary Experiments with Graft Size

The effect of graft size upon the host immune system was first studied by Medawar (1944) in the rabbit. Mention has already been made of the fact that in the conventional graft–host relationship a small allograft (low-dosage graft) has a longer survival time than a standard size allograft (high-dosage graft; see page xviii). Taken comprehensively, the histologic appearance showing the course of vascularization, infiltrative inflammatory reaction, and epithelial activity are quite similar in the two grafts. Because the low-dosage grafts survive longer, the evolution of such grafts extends beyond the proliferation phase and into the period of hair formation, accompanied by advanced retrograde differentiation of the blood vessels and epithelium of the graft epidermis and pilosebaceous units. Inflammatory and vascular proliferation are slower to develop and are not as obvious as in high-dosage grafts. Since the sequence of events leading to the rejection of low- and high-dosage allografts, as described in detail by Medawar (1944), is similar to that already reviewed in Chapter 2, no further comments are needed here. As stated by Medawar, the inverse relationship between the dosage of the grafted tissue and the length of its survival is not distinctly defined. In formulating his theory of acquired immunity, Medawar (1944, 1945) maintained that, due to the maximum amount of antigens released by the larger quantity of donor skin in a high-dosage graft, the immunologic mechanism attains its maximum strength and thereby reduces the period of graft survival in comparison to low-dosage grafts.

Medawar's findings were subsequently confirmed by Lehrfeld and Taylor (1953) in the rat. As evidenced by stereomicroscopy, although there is a significant difference in the survival time of different size grafts, the sequential vascular changes from the time of reestablished blood circulation to the time of allograft destruction are similar to those described previously by Taylor and Lehrfeld (1953), with the exception of some differences in the timing of events. Lehrfeld and Taylor (1953) found in the rat, as did Medawar (1944) in the adult rabbit, that the extent of the vascular proliferation and subsequent return to a more normal vascular pattern depend largely upon the timing of the graft rejection. On the basis of their experimental results, Lehrfeld and Taylor (1953) supported the acquired immunity hypothesis of allograft rejection, as proposed by Medawar (1944).

Edgerton and Edgerton (1955) and Edgerton *et al.* (1957), using the transparent mouse chamber technique, were unable to find any evidence of a dosage phenomenon.

Zotikov *et al.* (1960), in a series of experiments in rats, evaluated the reaction to the transplantation of massive skin allografts representing one-third of the body surface of the recipient. As mentioned in the Introduction, they discovered that the large graft survived longer than its smaller counterparts (Fig. 48). In a subsequent study, Zotikov and Urinson (1962) reexam-

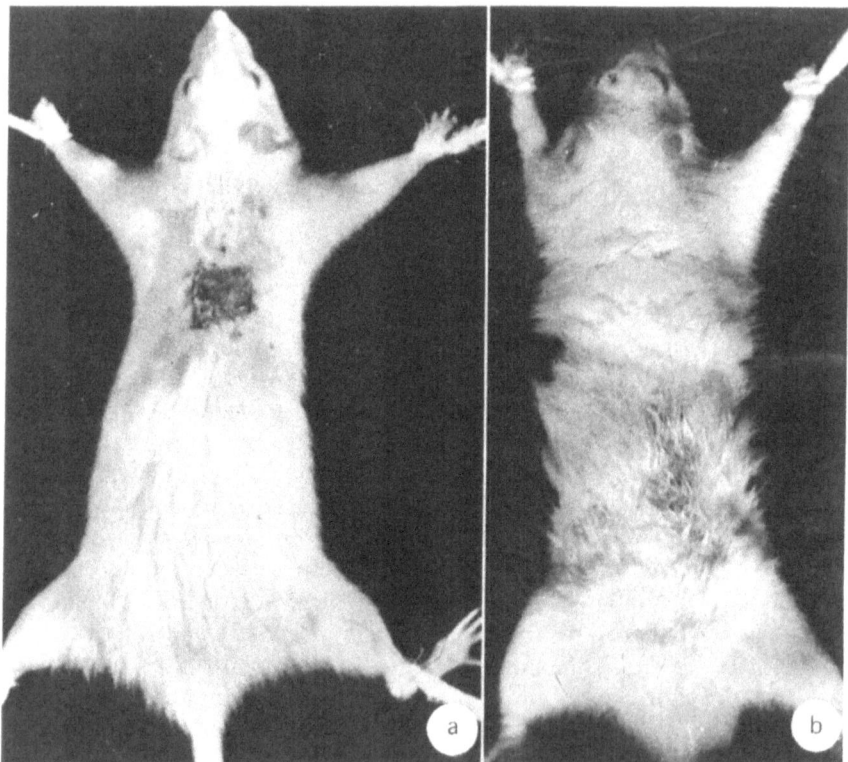

Fig. 48 a and b. Comparison of survival of large and small allografts in the rat. **a.** Small allograft on rat 2 weeks after operation. The allograft has withered and died. **b.** Large allograft on rat 8 months after operation. The allograft has survived. Zotikov, Budik, and Puza (1960) Ann. N.Y. Acad. Sci. 87:166.

ined the dosage phenomenon and confirmed the previous findings. The clinical status and the condition of the circulating blood were employed as diagnostic criteria in both series of experiments in the assessment of viability, behavior, and survival times of the grafts. However, the investigators did not explain nor specify the tests employed for establishing the state of circulation or the vascular events associated with the rejection response.

Other Experimental Studies

Gross inspection and occasional histology were used by Calnan and Kulatilake (1962) to assess the behavior and eventual fate of a skin allograft in rats. As stated by the authors, a surviving graft is "pinkish, soft, quiet, and clean," whereas a graft that fails to survive is "pale or brown, firm, and odorous." Basing their conclusions on these criteria of survival, Calnan and Kulatilake reported that grafts of massive dosage survived significantly longer than the smaller controls, confirming the findings of Zotikov et al. (1960). Furthermore, some of the large grafts surviving at 18 days exhibited patches of healthy epithelium as demonstrated by histology (Fig. 49). Although three possible theories—the formation of slough, antibody response, and method of assessment—were offered in attempts to explain prolonged survival, the authors admitted that none seems to be entirely satisfactory.

Further evidence of prolonged graft survival has been found by Converse, Siegel, and Ballantyne (1962, 1963) in the rat (Fig. 50a). They followed the sequence of vascular patterns occurring in skin allografts of massive dosage through a film of mineral oil under a stereomicroscope, using the diagnostic method of evaluation of Taylor and Lehrfeld (1953, 1955). On stereomicroscopic examination, the rate of blood flow is generally seen to be normal throughout the graft vascular system by the third or fourth day after grafting; the dilation of vessels noted during the first few days progressively subsides, and the vessels resume the pattern of normal skin until just before the rejection reaction. The earliest evidence of immune attack against massive donor tissue is manifested by the slowing down of blood flow and eventual hemal stasis, rapidly followed by capillary degeneration and vascular disruption. Many such grafts undergoing the process of immune rejection appear to be "melting away" (Fig. 50b). The melting away pattern occurs cyclically, characterized by a series of small periodic hemorrhages, followed by a slow undermining replacement by the host at several sites along the graft margins, giving the graft an appearance of being nipped. Severely burned patients with extensive loss of skin cover have been observed to display a similar rejection pattern in their allografts. It was suggested that antigenic overloading of the immune system in the rat host by the massive graft is responsible for prolonged survival. In contrast, in the burned patient the diminished immune response is the reason the graft can survive for a prolonged period.

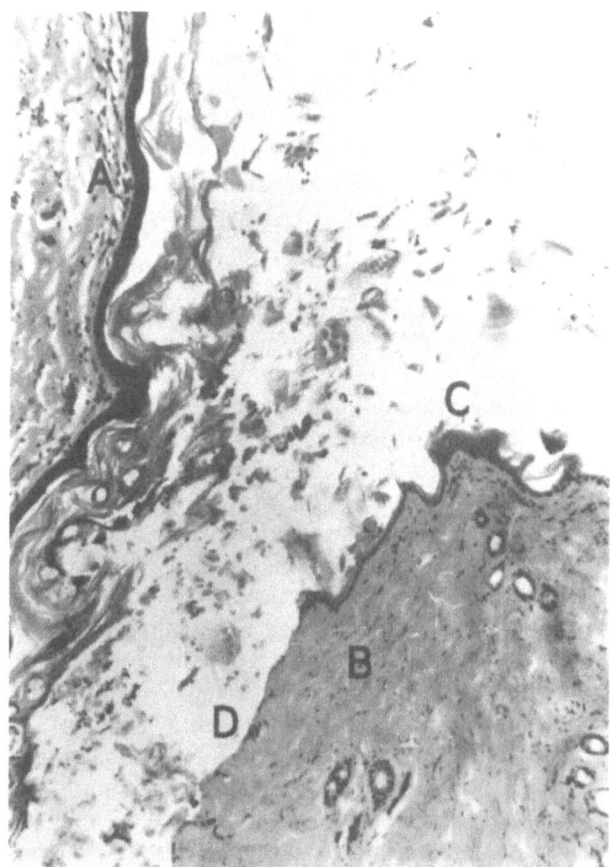

Fig. 49. Histologic section of massive allograft at 18 days showing graft–host junction A, normal skin with deeply stained epithelium and marked keratin (cuticle) formation; B, allograft dermis showing no infiltration of cells, and an apparently normal appearance; C, island of epithelium which stains a little less well than normal with hematoxylin but whose cells appear normal; D, allograft denuded of epithelium. H & E. ×100. Calnan and Kulatilake (1962) Br. J. Plast. Surg. 15:341.

These findings of protracted survival of massive skin grafts in the rat are at variance with the findings of Matter, Chambler, Lewis, and Blocker (1963) in similar animals. They claimed that prolonged survival could not be obtained with an increase in the size of the donor skin and it was suggested that graft acceptance is associated with histocompatibility rather than with quantity of tissue. Although the clinical appearance of the grafted tissue was examined every second day and punch biopsies (Fig. 51) were obtained 5 days after grafting and every 3 days thereafter, detailed descriptions of such

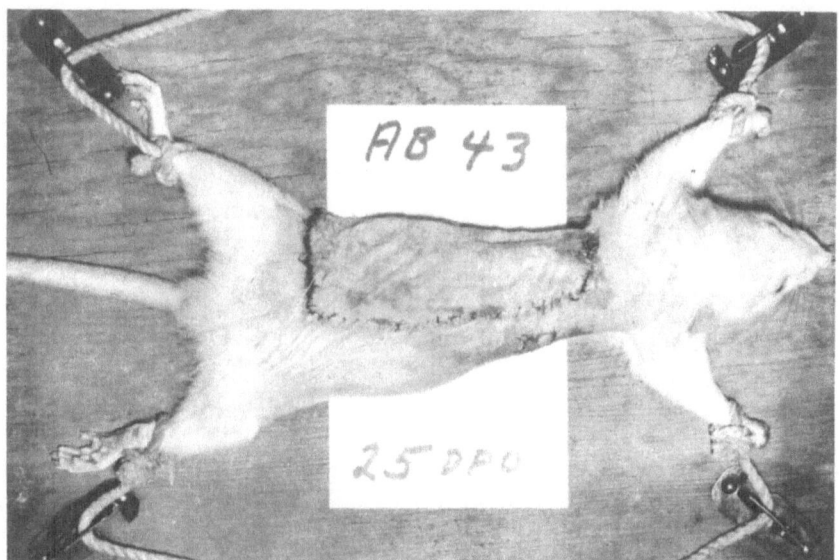

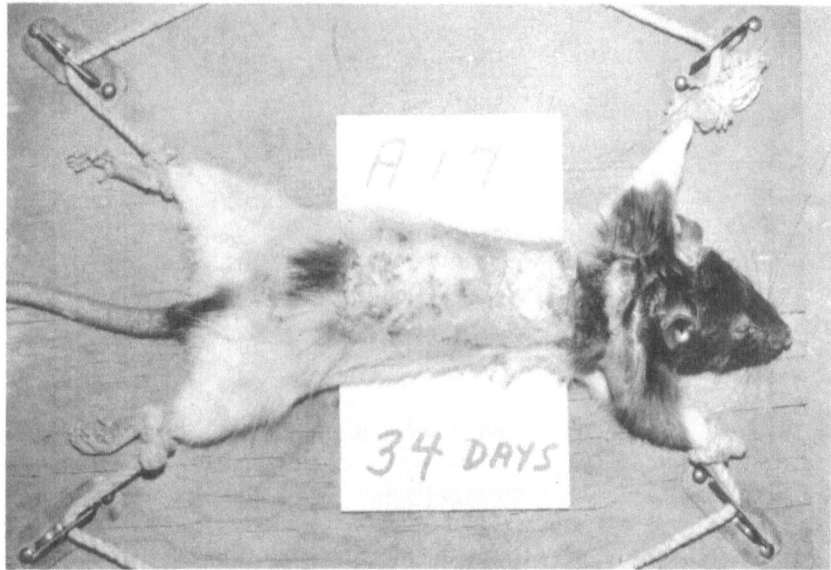

Fig. 50 a and b. Gross appearance of large skin allograft in the rat after prolonged survival. **a.** Note the normal appearance of the massive graft 25 days after transplantation. **b.** By 34 days after transplantation the graft is undergoing the process of "melting away," a mode of slow rejection observed in several large allografts. Converse, Siegel, and Ballantyne (1963) Plast. Reconstr. Surg. 31:9, © (1963) The Williams & Wilkins Co., Baltimore.

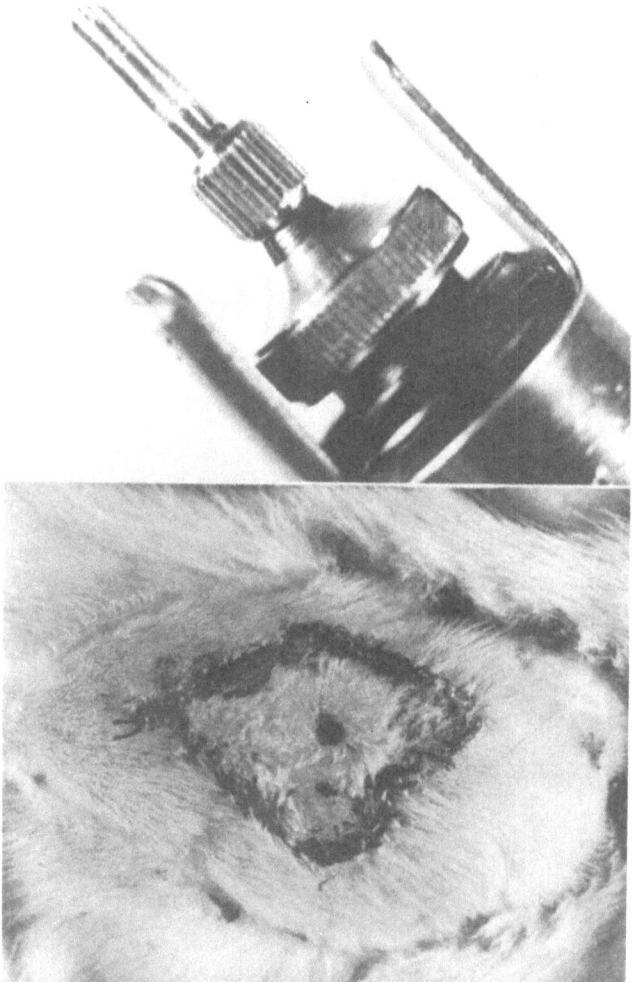

Fig. 51 a and b.   Punch biopsy technique. **a.** Drill for punch biopsies. **b.** Biopsy from a small allograft. Matter, Chambler, Lewis, and Blocker (1963) Transplantation 1:157, © (1963) The Williams & Wilkins Co., Baltimore.

observations, with respect to the diagnostic criteria for evaluating the graft condition and survival time, were not provided in their report. In addition, the investigators appeared to have problems with the grafting techniques, as demonstrated by the failure of small control autografts to survive. In view of these omissions and problems, a review of their work is not feasible. This also applies to the study by Veith *et al.* (1966), who compared the reactivity of massive skin allografts in dogs, under azathioprine and azaserine immunosuppressive therapy with that of small control allografts in similarly treated animals. Moreover, untreated dogs with allogeneic tissue of comparable size were not included in this experiment.

The appearance of hemagglutinating and cytotoxic isoantibodies in the sera of rat recipients following massive skin allotransplantation was reported by Kapitchnikov, Ballantyne, and Stetson (1962) and Ballantyne and Stetson (1964). Because the antibody response to grafts of massive dosage appeared at the same time and to the same extent as that observed in smaller grafts, it was concluded that the prolongation in the survival of large grafts is not due to immunologic paralysis of the host generated by large doses of donor antigen.

A subsequent serologic study in the rat was undertaken by Rother, Rother, and Ballantyne (1967) in order to evaluate the effect of graft size upon the serum complement activity (C'). From their serologic data showing no appreciable effect of the dosage phenomenon of skin grafts on the pattern of the complement titers in sera of individual recipients, the authors concluded that the exhaustion or inactivation of the complement system was not the factor responsible for the increased survival of large grafts.

Preliminary attempts were undertaken by Lapp and Bliss (1966) and Lappé, Graff, and Snell (1969) to evaluate the relationship between the size and survival time of skin allografts in mice incompatible at weak histocompatibility loci (H-1, H-3, or H-7) rather than the strong H-2 locus. It was determined that the survival times of skin allografts with weak incompatibility significantly improve with a progressive increase in the graft size. Lapp and Bliss attributed the prolongation of graft survival with the increase in graft size to the induction of immune tolerance, whereas Lappé, Graff, and Snell concluded that it may be a function of the target size alone.

Zanella, Reif, Buenviaje, Asakuma, and Deterling (1968) investigated the relationship between the size and survival time of full-thickness skin allografts exchanged between inbred strains of mice differing at the H-2 histocompatibility locus. Four different sizes of skin grafts—minute (0.3 × 0.3 cm), small (1.3 × 1.3 cm), large (1.5 × 3.0 cm), and massive (30–40% of the total body surface)—were evaluated in this experiment. The behavior and survival time of each graft were assessed by the diagnostic methods of visual and tactile inspection; a graft was considered to be rejected when 90% of the grafted skin became necrotic. It was determined that the survival times of allografts are significantly prolonged with an increase in the size of the donor tissue. The finding of Zanella and associates (1968) that minute allografts survived for shorter periods of time than small and large grafts are at sharp variance with the previous reports by Medawar (1944, 1945), Lehrfeld and Taylor (1953), Zotikov et al. (1960), and McKhann and Berrian (1961).

According to Zanella et al. (1968), their data showing 2–2.5 times longer survival times for massive allografts than small grafts in mice are consistent with the observations of Zotikov et al. (1960), Converse et al. (1962, 1963), Ballantyne, Siegel, and Kapitchnikov (1962), Ballantyne, Siegel, and Converse (1963), Ballantyne and Stetson (1964), and Rother *et al.* (1967) in the rat. It was suggested that there are three possible factors responsible for the decreased survival of minute allografts and the prolonged survival of massive grafts: (1) a nonspecific factor, such as a stress reaction produced by operative and postoperative trauma; (2) a depression of the immunologic reaction for the specific type of skin graft, similar to that previously proposed by Converse *et al.* (1962, 1963) to explain the survival of massive grafts; and (3) a nonspecific factor dependent upon the relationship between the graft size and the cellular dynamics associated with the rejection response.

The response of recipient mice to skin allografts varying in size from 1 to 8 cm² was subsequently reported by Gotjamanos (1970). Four sizes of full-thickness suprapannicular grafts—small (1 cm²), medium (4 or 4.5 cm²), large (6 cm²), and massive (8 cm²)—were exchanged across strong H-2 histocompatibility barriers between four inbred strains of mice. Similar size autografts and isografts were also prepared to serve as comparative controls. The macroscopic appearance of all in situ iso-, auto-, and allografts was observed, recorded, and correlated with the microscopic appearance.

In general outline, for the first 3–4 days after transplantation, regardless of the graft dosage and the actual source of the donor tissue, all grafts developed a deep pink color, indicating a hypervascular response in the graft bed; this hypervascularity then subsided. Whereas hair growth and normal skin appearance were evident in the autografts and isografts (Fig. 52a) at 15–16 days, most allografts exchanged across different H-2 loci acquired a gray or pale yellow-brown coloration by 6–7 days, with progression to a definite brown in the next 2–3 days (Fig. 52b). At this stage the surface of the allografts became very dry, following which numerous pitted areas soon appeared, exposing the underlying moist dermis. These changes, confirmed by microscopy, were variable among all allografts at 7 days; they became more prominent in massive and large grafts during the following few days.

It was concluded that in each of three different donor–recipient combinations used the mean survival time of massive skin allografts exceeded that of small grafts by 2–3 days, the difference being highly statistically significant by the standard analysis of variance techniques. However, the experimental evidence of Gotjamanos (1970) in mice does not seem to substantiate the finding of Zanella and associates (1968) in similar animals that massive grafts survive twice as long as small ones. The diminished immune response to a massive skin allograft was attributed by Gotjamanos (1970) to a combination of two possible mechanisms: a severe surgical trauma and a cellular response by the graft recipient sufficient to destroy and replace the foreign tissue. He also was of the opinion that the discrepancies between his findings and the previously reported findings and conclusions with regard to the graft size and its viability were due to different diagnostic assay procedures in the assessment of the graft survival time.

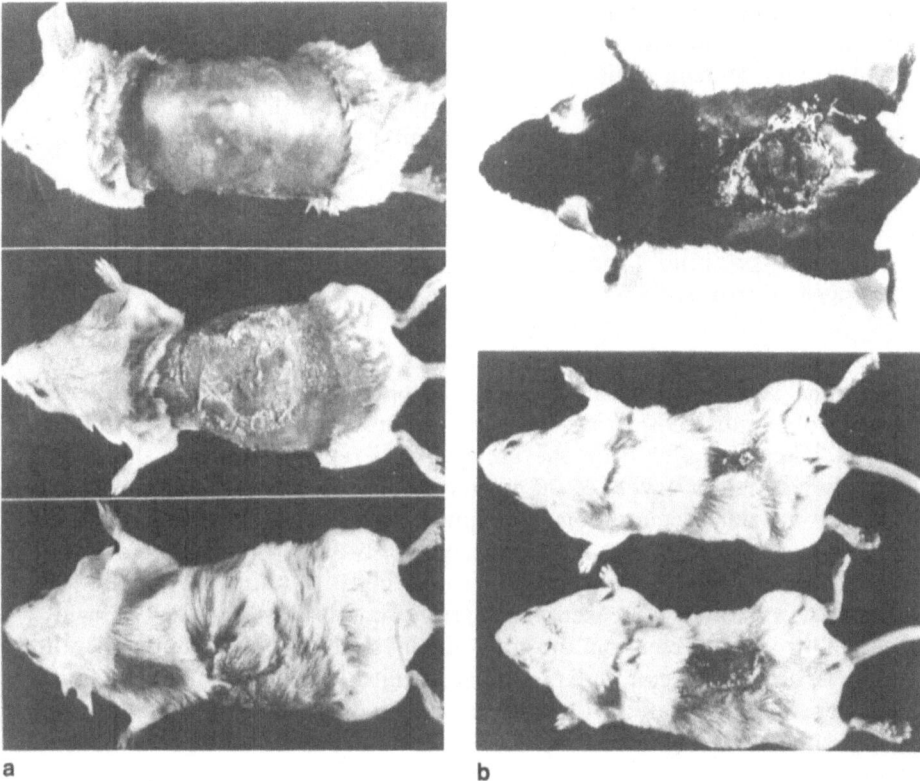

a   b

Fig. 52 a and b.   Fate of massive grafts transplanted across strong H-2 barriers in mice. **a.** Massive isograft. *Top:* 2 days after grafting. *Middle:* 15 days after grafting; the isograft shows the first evidence of continued hair growth. *Bottom:* 24 days after grafting; hair length and density have been almost restored to normal. **b.** Massive allografts. These grafts were originally the same size as the isograft shown in panel a. *Top:* C57 Black/6 mouse bearing remnants of AKR graft at 15 days; rejection of this graft had occurred at 11 days. *Bottom:* Balb/C mice with remnants of CBA grafts at 22 days; both of these grafts had been rejected at 10 days. Gotjamanos (1970) Aust. J. Exp. Biol. Med. Sci. 48:1.

In 1974 Guthy *et al.* studied the course of vascular and morphologic patterns in large full-thickness skin grafts in the guinea pig by means of combined assay procedures, visual inspection, stereomicroscopy, and histology (see page 24). They were unable to observe any evidence of tissue adherence at the graft–host junction, graft vascularization with hemal circulation, and tissue viability of large grafts. They attributed the lack of vascularization and early loss of viability in the massive grafts to intercepted vascularization resulting from a combination of mechanical and technical factors, followed by immunologic factors. Thus, the authors doubted the validity of the previous experiments of Converse, Ballantyne, Siegel, Rother, and Stetson which showed that massive skin allografts survive transplantation procedures, become vascularized, with strong stereomicroscopic evidence of active blood flow, and alter the immune responses in the host to grafts.

Effect of Specially Treated Host Beds on the Survival of Massive Skin Grafts

Working with rats, Ballantyne *et al.* (1962) studied the effect of artificially relocating and redistributing the blood supply in the host bed on the sequence of events leading to the rejection of massive skin allografts. Following excision of the skin on the dorsum of a recipient animal, the highly vascularized lateral layers of the panniculus carnosus were folded over the sparsely vascular region along the spinal cord and secured together with interrupted sutures. Compared to massive grafts on untreated beds, grafts of similar size placed on surgically treated beds were more rapidly vascularized, exhibited increased vascularity, and survived 6–7 days longer.

At the time of rejection, the grafts manifested signs of rejection over the entire tissue and did not undergo the premonitory breakdown in the midline area generally associated with grafts placed on intact beds. In massive grafts that had been transplanted to intact beds, a few days prior to graft rejection there was usually a complete cessation of blood flow, capillary breakdown, and vascular disruption in the dorsomedian aspect of the graft, followed by discoloration, induration, and necrosis. In contrast to this, due to the improved blood supply in the area where it is normally deficient, there was no premature discoloration or necrosis in the central part of the massive grafts that had been transferred to specially treated beds.

Experiments with Massive Skin Xenografts

Ballantyne *et al.* (1969) transplanted full-thickness massive skin grafts from rabbit flanks and auricles to prepared recipient sites in a series of 30 rats; an additional 30 rats bearing small grafts of rabbit skin served as comparative controls. Periodic gross and stereomicroscopic examinations showed that massive grafts survived twice as long as the small control grafts. In addition, strong tissue adhesion between the graft and host and the reestablishment of a major definitive vasculature with brisk blood flow were observed in both massive and small grafts. However, the process of vascularization was delayed in the massive grafts until 5–7 days after transplantation, whereas the small grafts were rapidly vascularized and a rapid blood flow was already evident in most grafts by 3–4 days. In addition, there were appreciable differences in the manner in which the two different sizes of rabbit skin grafts were destroyed by the immune system of the rat recipient.

In massive grafts, the earliest stereomicroscopic indication of the onset of rejection was the distention and cessation of blood flow in a few graft vessels, but without any evidence of vascular disruption. This was indicated grossly by the appearance of small brownish spots with no particular pre-dilection as to the site on the graft surface. The spots subsequently increased in density and size until the graft survival end points were characterized by the complete confluence of these discolored areas occupying the entire extent of the graft. This event was accompanied by a significant loss in tissue turgor and elasticity. While this pattern of chronic rejection occurred in most of the massive grafts, other xenografts underwent a peculiar mode of en bloc rejection, which was reflected by discoloration appearing suddenly at a margin and spreading rapidly over the entire surface.

These findings were in distinct contrast to those observed in small skin xenografts, in which a rapid and violent process of rejection, which usually occurred 6–7 days after grafting, was characterized by the complete coales-cence of discolored areas over the entire tissue surface, tissue hardening, and vascular disruption.

As interpreted by Ballantyne *et al.* (1969), in massive rabbit skin grafts transplanted to rats, certain tissue areas that are the first to receive a blood supply from the host may also be the sites of the earliest antigen–antibody reaction, whereas other parts, not yet vascularized, are temporarily toler-ated. This assumption appears to be supported by the stereomicroscopic findings that the localized areas of tissue destruction, as indicated grossly by brown spots, were found in the immediate vicinity of graft tissue showing normal blood flow. As the vascularization process continued throughout the remaining graft dermis, more of the tissue thus became subject to the immunologic response by the host. The en bloc pattern of rejection observed in some grafts may have reflected the simultaneous vascularization over the entire graft, with the result that the graft was completely rejected within 1–2 days.

Summary

There is considerable evidence from most of the studies reviewed here that massive skin allografts in rats survive longer than smaller grafts. Prolonged survival of massive grafts was assessed by periodic gross and stereomicro-scopic observations, correlated with occasional histologic evidence. The results show that, apart from the difference in the rejection time of massive and smaller control grafts, the appearance, behavior, and sequence of vascu-lar events from the time of transplantation to the rejection period are remarkably similar in the massive and smaller grafts. Despite several serologic studies, the nature of the mechanisms responsible for the temporary tolerance and delayed rejection of large grafts has not yet been elucidated.

Evidence of delayed immunologic responses to grafts of massive dosage in a different animal species, the mouse, has been provided by Zanellas and associates (1968) and Gotjamanos (1970). However, there are sharp differences of opinion concerning the effect of graft size upon the immune system of the host in the rat (Matter *et al.* 1963), dog (Veith *et al.* 1966), and guinea pig (Guthy *et al.* 1974).

Chapter 6

Behavior of Preserved Skin Grafts in Their Hosts

This chapter is concerned with experimental and clinical observations of the biologic events that occur in preserved skin grafts after transplantation to recipients. The various types of preservative techniques, the duration and temperature of graft storage, and the diagnostic assay procedures for assessing the condition and eventual fate of preserved skin grafts following transplantation are also briefly described.

The discussion will first center on the indications for the clinical application of preserved skin grafts as biologic dressings or temporary cover in patients. It has long been recognized that an available and adequate source of preserved skin grafts is of major importance in reconstructive surgery, especially in the treatment of burns or extensive loss of skin due to mechanical trauma. Preserved skin autografts are useful in multiple-stage reconstructive surgical procedures. The survival of the extensively burned patient can be assured only after successful coverage of the raw areas resulting from the full-thickness destruction of the skin. Skin allografts, although eventually rejected by the host, serve as a vital and often lifesaving temporary cover, especially in the treatment of burns.

The prospect of covering extensive skin loss with fresh or preserved skin xenografts as a temporary biologic dressing until permanent repair with autografts can be instituted has attracted many investigators and surgeons during the past half century. The application of bovine fetal skin (Silvetti, Cotton, Bryne, Berrian, and Menendez 1957; Sokolic, Farpour, Ulin, and Howard 1959) and pigskin (Eastwood 1961; Song *et al.* 1966) as temporary covers for large skin defects in humans has elicited considerable interest because they are readily available as commercial preparations. Apart from alleviating pain (Pandya and Zarem, 1974) and reducing bacterial counts in the granulation tissue (Eade 1958; Song *et al.* 1966; Switzer *et al.* 1966), fetal calf and porcine skin xenografts have been of some use in enhancing the early appearance of healthy and highly vascular granulation tissue in the recipient bed (O'Donoghue and Zarem 1971). Furthermore, these grafts do not provoke any significant immunologic reactions in the host (Pate 1954; Rogers *et al.* 1957; Sokolic *et al.* 1959; Song *et al.* 1966).

For many years the problem of developing satisfactory methods for preserving skin in the live state at temperatures near or above freezing and storing it in the frozen state has been a subject of considerable interest. Clinically, the freeze-drying process consists of (1) procurement of skin from patients, volunteers, or cadavers under sterile conditions, (2) rapid freezing of the tissue to low temperatures, (3) dehydration (drying) of skin from the frozen state, (4) long-term storage of the freeze-dried skin grafts at room temperature and, (5) rehydration at the time of clinical use.

In a comprehensive review of approximately 200 reports, Perry (1966) described and discussed the advantages and difficulties associated with three methods of skin storage—nutrient media refrigeration, preservation of skin in the frozen state, and freeze-drying of skin for storage at room temperature. He also reviewed the clinical and experimental studies on the effect of each preservative method on the behavior and survival of skin grafts.

Storage at Temperatures Above Freezing

Mammalian tissues, excised and kept at body or room temperature, become anoxemic and necrotic after a period of 48 hours; the fact that such changes can be retarded by oxygenation or by chilling is common knowledge. It would appear, therefore, that tissue metabolism (of oxygen, nutrients, and waste products) must be ensured and the rate of metabolism retarded by a reduction in temperature in order to keep isolated tissue alive. Baronio first demonstrated in 1804 that the viability of mammalian skin can be maintained temporarily. After excising full-thickness pieces of skin from sheep, he stored them at room temperature for short periods up to 1 hour and then successfully employed them as autografts.

The simplest method of storing split-thickness skin grafts is by suturing the grafts to the donor site. Shepard (1972) has shown that skin grafts can be stored without complications on their donor sites and transferred at the bedside without the need for an anesthetic for a period of up to 10 days. The technique lends itself to delayed grafting whenever hemostasis is incomplete or there is an avascular recipient bed.

Early Clinical and Experimental Studies

Wentscher, in 1903, appears to have been the first to report successful storage of skin by refrigeration, as demonstrated by the survival of human skin autografts. The grafts had been either wrapped with moistened gauze or immersed in saline solution and preserved at temperatures near 0°C for periods of 7 or 12 days.

In 1912 Carrel stored segments of skin from a dog in tubes containing petrolatum at temperatures varying between −1° and 7°C for 1–10 days; these grafts could be transplanted with the same degree of success as freshly excised skin grafts. Carrel found that Ringer's solution was inferior to petrolatum as a preservative medium; he also reported that fresh human skin grafts treated similarly healed in place as well as freshly excised nontreated grafts.

Webster, in 1944, described his successful experiments with fresh human skin wrapped in plioform, over which he placed several layers of vaseline gauze, which in turn was covered with two sterile towels for storage at approximately 4°C. He stated that, in a number of cases, such tissues had survived a storage period of 3 weeks when applied as skin autografts to suitable recipient sites (Fig. 53).

Survival of autogenous human skin for longer periods was observed by Matthews (1945). He wrapped the tissue in a piece of tulle-gras, surrounded it in turn with gauze tightly wrung out of saline solution, and kept the wrapped tissues in a screw-capped bottle in a refrigerator at 3°–6°C. The rate of vascularization, the pattern of color changes, the texture and pliability, and the gross and histologic appearance of the refrigerated skin when applied as autografts after storage periods of 3–8 weeks were similar to those of the freshly excised grafts.

Employing a procedure similar to that of Matthews, except that the excised skin was not wrapped with the saline-soaked gauze, Flatt (1948) obtained satisfactory results following a storage period of 2 months.

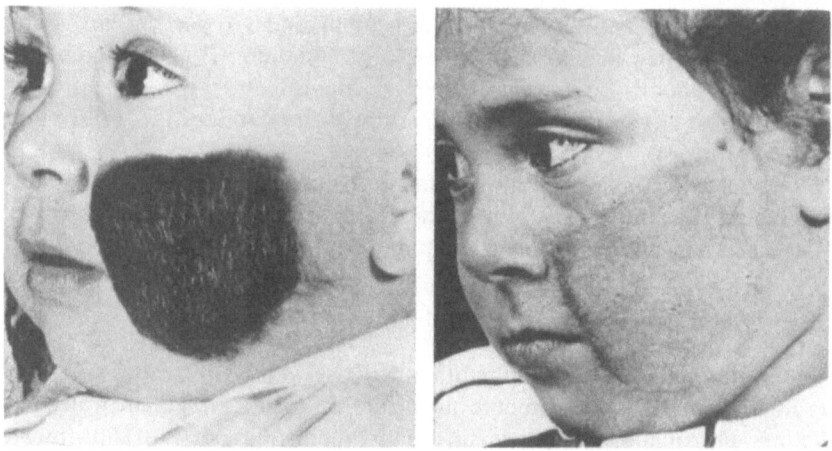

Fig. 53 a and b. In this case the skin graft was refrigerated and the operation terminated because of the precarious condition of the patient. The skin was applied 4 days later. **a.** Condition before operation. **b.** Condition 3 years after operation. Webster (1944) Ann. Surg. 120:431.

Subsequent Studies in Humans and Animals

Other investigators strove to determine the optimum conditions for the survival of skin stored in a similar temperature range. Hanks and Wallace (1949), experimenting with rabbit skin, cited the superiority of 10% serum to mineral oil as a storage medium. They based their assessment of the viability of stored skin on tissue culture techniques following storage at 0° and at 6° to 8°C. The superior survival of the serum-treated skin grafts was attributed to the nutrients provided by this medium as well as the buffering action against acids liberated by tissue metabolism. Marrangoni (1950) and Allgöwer and Blocker (1952) confirmed the superiority of dilute serum as a medium for the storage of rabbit and human skin grafts at refrigerator temperatures.

These experiments indicated that the best conditions for the storage of skin grafts at temperatures above freezing include (1) immersion in a medium consisting of 10–30% serum in a balanced salt solution, (2) the presence of air, and (3) storage at a temperature of about 5°C. The viability of excised skin under these conditions may be sustained for at least 1 week, and at most for 2 months. The viability of the stored tissue progressively declines during the storage period, however, and prolonged storage introduces the risk of less than complete survival.

Modifications of dilute sera, physiologic solutions, or tissue culture media as well as other various protective agents for graft storage above 0°C were described by many subsequent investigators (Hyatt, Turner, Bassett, Pate, and Sawyer 1952; Medawar 1954; Pepper 1954; Georgiade, Peschel, Georgiade, and Brown 1956; Perry, Evans, Young, Earle, and Hyatt 1957; Gresham, Perry, and Thompson 1963; Raju and Grogan 1969b). Silicone fluid (Ballantyne, Hawthorne, Rees, and Seidman 1971) and deuterated medium (Wandall 1972) were tested in the rat and pig, respectively, as possible protective media for the storage of skin grafts at refrigerator temperatures.

The sum of the information obtained from the experiments leads to the conclusion that the upper limit of the storage time of skin is 8 weeks, or in some cases an even shorter time span.

Biochemical Studies

The first biochemical investigation of preserved skin grafts was that of De Stefano in 1959. He directed his attention to the enzymatic activities of alkaline phosphatase and trypsin occurring in allografts of full-thickness rabbit skin that had been placed in a very small quantity of toluene and kept at 2°C for 8 hours. From the quantitative estimates in tissue samples immediately prior to and at time intervals after transplantation, the phosphatase activity of the skin allografts following short-term storage was not as great as that in freshly prepared control grafts. The loss of enzymatic activity was correlated with an increase in the survival time of stored grafts when compared to that of the normal and untreated grafts. Consequently, De Stefano inferred that the decline in enzymatic levels from the effects of storage is closely associated with a reduction in tissue antigenicity as reflected by the prolonged survival of the grafts. Unlike alkaline phosphatase, there was no demonstrable evidence that trypsin was present in either control or stored transplants.

Effects of storage on the succinic dehydrogenase activity and the viability of guinea pig skin were assessed by Donaldson, Payne, and Hershey in 1960. The histochemical demonstration of succinic dehydrogenase and the levels of its activity in the control and preserved skin was achieved by in vitro incubation of selected tissue samples in physiologic solutions containing tetrazolium salts as reduction indicators. At the end of incubation the tetrazolium is reduced to formazan and is deposited in the tissue as a water-soluble red pigment which is extracted and then allowed to stand overnight in methyl cellosolve. Following this, the optical density (OD) of the solution, already stained orange by the extracted material, is measured with a Beckman DU spectrophotometer at 490 μm. The intensity of the succinic dehydrogenase activity, calculated from the deposition of formazan produced by tetrazolium, is expressed as units of optical density of formazan per milligram of tissue. As explained by the investigators, if the amount of succinic dehydrogenase in the skin is equal to or exceeds 50 OD units, all grafts survive the preservation procedures and transplantation is confirmed by a reversed crop of hair growth; whereas below the level of 50 OD units, less than one-half of the grafts are successful. Accordingly, the grafts that had been stored at 4°C for 6 days retained their original viability when subsequently autografted. When the storage period was extended to 9 days, the viability of the stored skin rapidly and progressively declined, and when storage was prolonged to 13 days, all grafts failed to survive the transplantation.

Studies on Bovine Embryo Skin Grafts

By means of gross and histologic observations, Sokolic and co-workers (1959) found, in dogs and humans, that after lyophilization or storage in physiologic saline solution at 4°C bovine embryo skin adhered well to its host bed during the first 2 days and provided an effective coverage for a period of 4–5 days. However, the xenografts showed no clear evidence of vascularization and elicited a more violent polymorphonuclear cell infiltration at the donor–host interface than that of an allograft reaction. Usually by the end of 6 days there was complete separation of the graft from its bed and the graft appeared completely shriveled. During this experiment the measurements of circulating antibodies by hemagglutination techniques and the passive cutaneous anaphylaxis test revealed no demonstrable evidence of local or systemic hypersensitivity induced by the bovine grafts in the recipient.

Summary

Marrangoni (1950) recommended storage of skin autografts in 10% serum in a standard refrigerator. Skin grafts can be wrapped in a saline-soaked sponge and stored in a sterile Petri dish. As shown by Feller and DeWeese (1958), human skin covered with a small piece of sponge moistened with Hartman's solution and stored in a glass jar in a refrigerator at 4°C remains viable for up to 23 days. After 14 days of storage in saline, skin graft respiratory activity is halved (J. C. Lawrence 1972). After 20 days skin cellular respiration ceases, and this effect corresponds with a progressive decrease in the clinical viability of skin stored in a refrigerator at 3°C over a 3-week period (Georgiade *et al.* 1956).

Despite the limitation imposed by the relatively short storage and reduced graft survival times, a simple and rapid short-term procedure for storing skin in a refrigerator appeals to clinicians. It permits immediate excision of skin from volunteers or cadavers, subsequent storage with a minimum of equipment, and availability for immediate application to a patient. In addition, these limitations have led to investigations of the preservation of skin in the frozen state at room temperatures. Skin allografts are also currently stored in a refrigerator for delayed skin grafting. Grafting is postponed for a few days if the recipient shows unusual bleeding that is difficult to control at the primary operation, if the operation cannot be completed because of the condition of the patient, or if an enhancement of the revascularization of the graft is desired (Šmahel 1971b).

Preservation by Freezing and Freeze-Drying

Injury to biologic systems preserved at low temperature has been attributed to the mechanical rupture and displacement of cytologic structures by growing ice crystals (Chambers and Hale 1932) and to the forces of expansion and contraction accompanying temperatures changes (for a review, see Luyet and Gehenio 1940). The failure to resume activities after freezing and drying has been attributed to changes in the concentration of electrolytes (Lovelock 1953) and salts by dehydration and the breakup of essential proteins and enzymes. These possibilities have been given consideration by many investigators who have attempted to reduce mechanical distortions and physicochemical changes within the cellular and fibrous structures by treating the skin with dilute sera, physiologic media, or other various protective agents prior to freezing and thawing.

In view of the fact that skin is composed of widely diversified types of cellular and fibrous constituents, Ballantyne and Converse, in 1966, undertook a review of various structural elements of the epidermis and dermis of normal skin at the cellular, subcellular, and molecular levels in an attempt to better understand possible changes occurring within the skin when frozen, thawed, and/or treated with cryoprotective agents. They expected that an increased knowledge of the response to freezing, drying, and storage would lead to the successful preservation of skin for medical purposes.

Storage of Mammalian Skin in the Frozen State

Early experimental evidence of the survival of mammalian skin was submitted by Mider and Morton in 1939; pieces of rat skin frozen to −50°C and then thawed were grafted subcutaneously. Their best results were obtained when the grafts were slowly frozen; the survival of some of the cells was evidenced by epithelial cyst formation and the presence of mitotic figures. Similar findings were observed in rat tissue frozen to −74°C, stored for 24 hours, thawed, and examined histologically 10 days after transplantation (compare Fig. 54b with a). Subsequently, Briggs and Jund (1944) made successful orthotopic transplantations of skin grafts in mice after the grafts were slowly frozen to −78.5°C, stored in dry ice for 1–2 days, and thawed. The successful application of frozen split-thickness autografts of human skin (Fig. 55a and b) that had been frozen to between −20° and −25°C and stored below −15°C for 1–61 days was described by Strumia and Hodge in 1945.

In 1950, Vanni, working with rabbits and guinea pigs, immersed skin autografts and allografts in the serum of the prospective recipients for the purposes of "biologic adaptation" and stored them at −3°C. Rabbits failed to accept their grafts, whereas 7 of 11 guinea pig grafts were successful; no adaptation was observed in any of the preserved allografts, which were eventually replaced by scar tissue. Billingham and Medawar (1952) concluded from their own studies that rabbit skin is quite resistant to damage by freezing and thawing and even to prolonged storage −79°C. Slow freezing and rapid thawing were found to be the least damaging to the graft.

The discovery by Polge, Smith, and Parkes (1949) that treatment with glycerol solution offered considerable protection to spermatozoa against the injury of freezing gave impetus to research on the effects of protective treatment with glycerol as well as ethylene glycol on the preservation of skin (Billingham and Medawar 1952; Keeley, Gomez, and Brown 1952; Taylor and Gerstner 1955). The action of glycerol protection against freezing was described by Lovelock (1953, 1954), who considered it as a buffer against the harmful concentration of salt, and also by Smith (1954).

Stereomicroscopic observations were made by Taylor, Gerstner, and Converse (1956) in order to follow the course of vascular changes in mammalian transplants preserved at temperatures below freezing. Revascularization

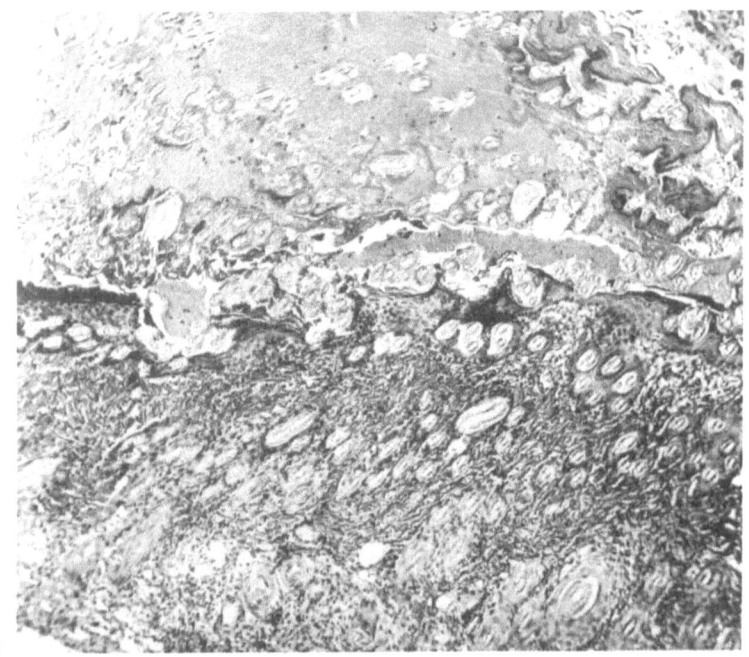

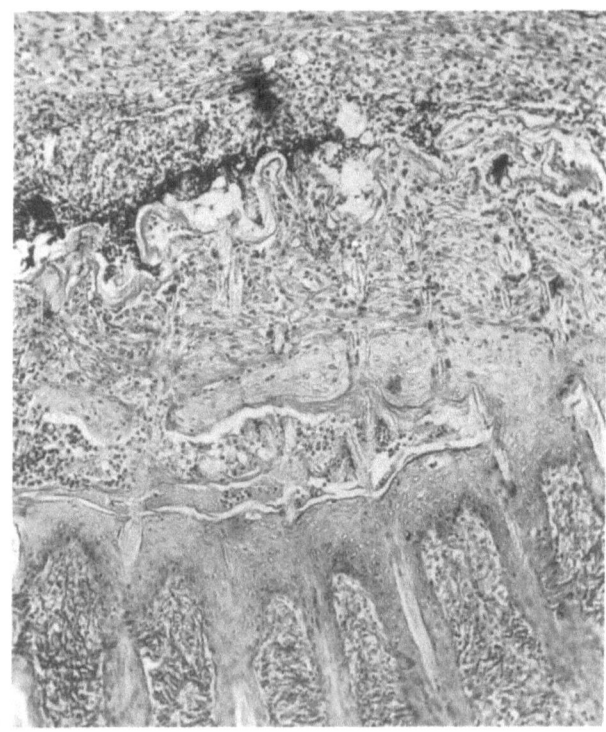

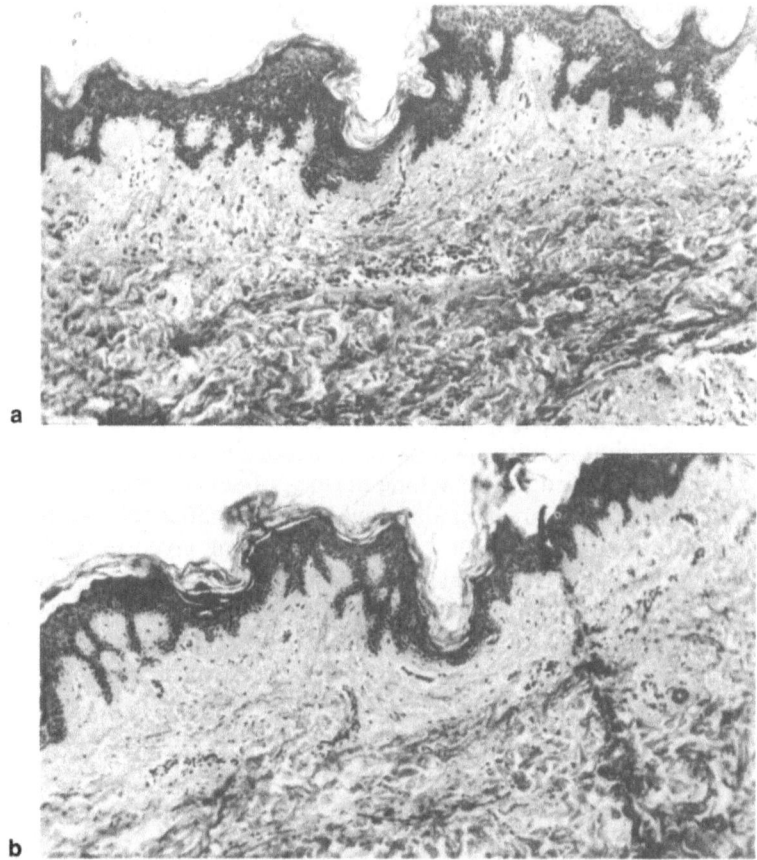

Fig. 55 a and b. Comparison of fresh and frozen human skin. **a.** Normal fresh skin. **b.** Skin frozen and preserved in the frozen state for 3 months. Strumia and Hodge (1945) Ann. Surg. 121:860.

Fig. 54 a and b *(Opposite).* Comparison of fresh and frozen and thawed rat skin grafts. **a.** Homologous subcutaneous transplant of normal unfrozen rat skin excised after 10 days. The upper part is the cyst. A layer of skin epithelium crosses the middle of the picture, below which the corium is seen, containing hair follicles and inflammatory cells. ×87. **b.** Homologous subcutaneous transplant of normal rat skin, frozen slowly to −74°C and immediately thawed, excised after 10 days. The upper part of the picture shows the granulation tissue of the host. Between this and the skin, in the lower part of the picture, lies a cyst filled with debris. ×104. Mider and Morton (1939) Am. J. Cancer 35:502.

was always delayed in frozen grafts, occurring as late as 5–7 days after grafting. In contrast, revascularization occurred within 3 days in untreated and normal skin grafts. The effect of the various freezing and thawing treatments and of various cryoprotective agents upon the viability and fate of the orthotopic skin grafts was correlated with the in vitro culture tests. The results were in agreement with the tissue culture experiments, showing a marked protective effect of pretreatment with glycerol and ethylene glycol. A sufficient number of cells survived in the protected and frozen grafts to form a grafted area with all the characteristics of normal skin.

Most grafts frozen without pretreatment were invaded by cells from the host site or were undergrown and cast off. Occasionally, however, living cells were observed adjacent to host tissue. This suggested that if the graft could be given an even more favorable environment than that offered by orthotopic treatment, a larger number of frozen cells might survive.

The skin of adult rabbits and chickens, according to Billingham (1961), can be very easily stored for very long periods of several months or more, provided that the grafts are first thoroughly impregnated for 1–2 hours at room temperature in a 15% by volume solution of glycerol in Ringer's solution. Following this treatment, the excess fluid is drained and the grafts are sealed in airtight stoppered glass vials. These containers are subsequently slowly frozen to −79°C. At the time of transplantation, it is necessary to accomplish the thawing of preserved tissue as rapidly as possible by immersing it in a 37°C water bath.

Experimenting with full-thickness rat skin, Santoni-Rugiu (1962) observed that the rate of survival of deep-frozen skin autografts stored for 14 days at −70°C was 40%. It was concluded that the reduced viability of deep-frozen allografts is responsible for their superiority to fresh allografts when grafted to recipient rats.

By using 15% glycerol in Ringer's solution as the cryoprotective medium, Bondoc and Burke (1971) showed that split-thickness skin obtained from guinea pigs, live human donors, or cadavers within 10 hours after death could be stored at −160°C with liquid nitrogen for up to 6 months. As shown by clinical findings and radiography with tritiated thymidine, there appeared to be no difference in the appearance of the graft vascularization and epidermal cell activity between the frozen, banked skin grafts and the freshly harvested grafts (Fig. 56a and b). According to J. C. Lawrence (1972), the metabolic activity of guinea pig ear skin and human split-thickness skin grafts treated with 15% glycerol and stored in liquid nitrogen for periods of up to 28 days was 60–70% of its original activity. Compared to 94% of freshly excised skin autografts, 84% of the preserved grafts survived transplantation.

Cryophylactic Action of Dimethyl Sulfoxide

The efficacy of dimethyl sulfoxide (DMSO) as a protective medium for skin storage at temperatures below freezing was evaluated by Lehr, Berggren,

a

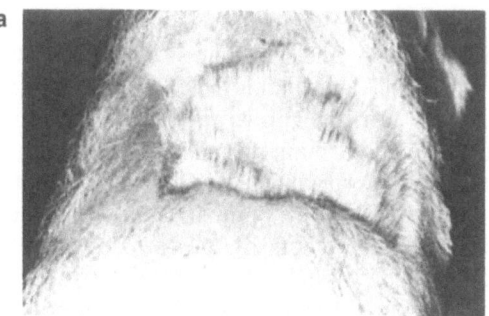

b

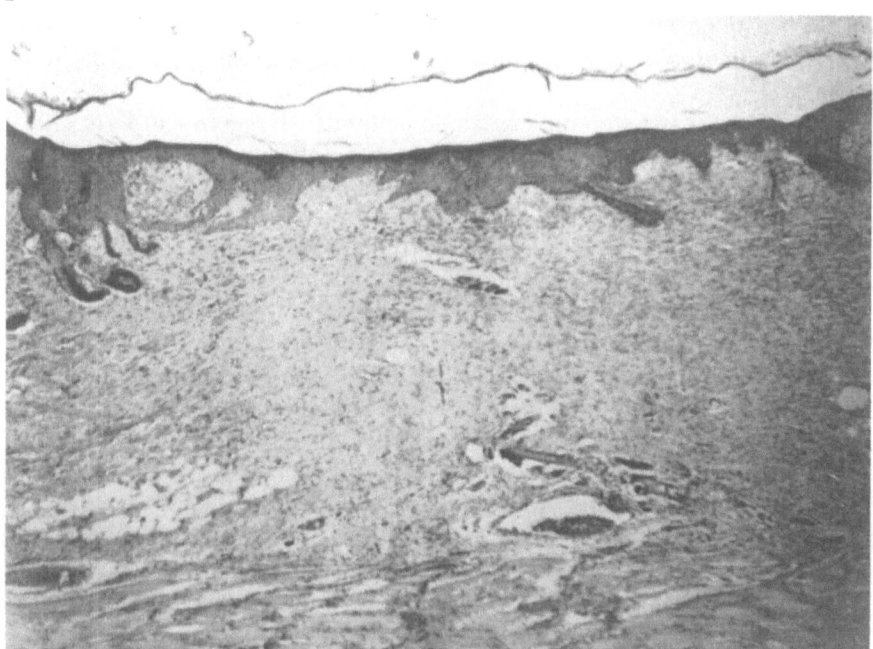

Fig. 56 a and b. Comparison of fresh and frozen guinea pig skin grafts. **a.** Split-skin autografts after transplantation. *Left:* fresh, unfrozen skin. *Right:* frozen graft 29 days after transplantation. **b.** Section taken from grafted frozen skin showing complete take including regeneration of hair follicles in the graft. Bondoc and Burke (1971) Ann. Surg. 174:371.

Lotke, and Coriell (1964) and by Barlyn, Berggren, and Lehr (1964). Although there have been reports on the noxious effects of DMSO, this compound in proper concentrations has been shown to protect mammalian skin against freezing injuries. Segments of split-thickness skin removed from the rat abdomen were impregnated with various cryophylactic media for 20–30 minutes at room temperature, stored at 4° to 7°C over various periods of time, and then autografted. Various rates of freezing and thawing were also evaluated. The reactivity and survival of each preserved rat skin autograft were assessed by gross and histologic examination; any graft that successfully maintained its normal appearance for more than 28 days was considered to have survived permanently. The preliminary data showed that under ideal conditions, glycerol and DMSO, in a concentration of 10% in either normal saline or serum, were comparable and seemed most effective in protecting grafts from the effects of the freezing and thawing process. Other findings indicated that skin could be successfully transplanted after a storage period of 7 days, whereas half of the autografts failed to retain tissue viability after 10 days of storage and none survived when stored for 14 days. Compared to the freezing rate, the thawing rate is considered to be more critical, and thawing should be accomplished rapidly in order to be successful.

Using gross and stereomicroscopic methods, Berggren and Lehr (1965) found that some human split-thickness autografts and allografts became effectively vascularized after treatment with 10% DMSO solution and storage in the frozen state for periods up to 608 days. If the grafts were not viable, they exhibited no evidence of vascularization and as a consequence became soft, white, and nonadherent.

In similar experiments with full-thickness autografts of mouse skin, Sherman (1965) found that both DMSO and glycerol protected tissues from injury by freezing and thawing. His technique consisted of immersing tissue segments in 5% or 15% by volume solutions of glycerol or DMSO in Ringer's solution for 1 hour at 22°C. The tissue was then frozen to −75°C at the rate of 1.3°C/minute, followed by thawing in 22°C Ringer's solution at the rate of 180°C/minute and transplantation. It was concluded that DMSO is at least as protective and toxic as glycerol and that the 5% solutions of DMSO and glycerol are less toxic and produce a greater post-thaw survival rate than the 15% solutions. Sherman (1965) also stressed the importance of pretreatment with protective media as a factor in freeze–thaw survival, as evidenced by a 22–55% loss of grafts due to treatment with DMSO or glycerol prior to freezing, not because of the freezing and thawing procedure.

Based on his experience with guinea pig ear skin and split-thickness human skin stored in liquid nitrogen for 2 days, J. C. Lawrence (1972) stated that 15% glycerol is superior to 15% DMSO as a cryoprotective agent; the latter has been found to be more toxic to skin after prolonged contact.

Studies on Porcine Skin Xenografts

In 1970 Rappaport, Pepino, and Dietrick cited histologic similarities between the frozen–irradiated and fresh refrigerated split-thickness porcine skin grafts placed on dogs and found no evidence of graft vascularization. Clinically, the porcine grafts provided an effective biologic dressing in the burn patient and an appreciable reduction in pain, particularly over second-degree burns.

Using the direct examination of blood vessels within the mouse transparent chamber, O'Donoghue and Zarem (1971) found that the preserved isografts are capable of inducing hyperemia and neovascularization in the recipient bed (Fig. 19a and b) and of becoming vascularized (Fig. 19c). Hyperemia appears in the host beds of the lyophilized grafts and the frozen–thawed grafts by 5 days after transplantation; but neovascularization occurs on days 7 and 8 in the respective host beds. The vascularization of the grafts is completely achieved by days 10 and 11, respectively. It is of interest to note that lyophilized grafts seem to be more effective in inducing host vascular budding and penetration into the lyophilized graft than are frozen–thawed grafts. Similar results were reported by Rogers and Converse (1958) in an earlier study using fresh and freeze-dried embryonic skin grafts transplanted to skin defects in man (see the section on the Evaluation of Freeze-Dried Skin Xenografts). With the same mouse chamber technique, Pandya and Zarem (1974) were not able to demonstrate vascularization in either the vacuum-dried or frozen xenografts of porcine split-thickness skin on mice during 15 days of observation.

Preservation of Freeze-Dried Skin at Room Temperature

Freeze-drying nearly satisfies the requirements of a preservative method since it maintains most of the structural details of cells and presumably leaves many of the proteins and enzymes of the tissue intact. The process involves the rapid freezing of the tissue by immersing it in liquid nitrogen or chilled isopentane. High-speed freezing reduces the mechanical distortion of the microscopic structure caused by the slow growth of ice crystals in and between the cells. This tissue is subsequently kept frozen while its water is removed from the solid state by sublimation. The dried tissue is usually sealed in a vacuum and stored at room temperature.

Histologic examination of the freeze-dried and rehydrated tissues has shown that the cytologic structure is best preserved when freezing is conducted very rapidly (Hoerr 1936). This is attributed to the fact that smaller ice crystals are formed in the tissues during rapid freezing than during slow freezing. The possibility of a correlation between the rate of freezing and the viability of frozen cells has been investigated by Breedis, Barnes, and Furth (1937), Snell and Cloudman (1943), Billingham and Medawar (1952), and Keeley et al. (1952).

Most investigators believe that lyophilized skin grafts do not contain vital cells. Webster (1944) cited the successful "take" of freeze-dried human autografts, but did not report the details of the method of drying or indications of the amount of water remaining in the skin at the end of lyophilization.

Clinical and Experimental Studies on Freeze-Dried Skin Grafts

Billingham and Medawar, in 1952, made a quantitative study of the ability of rabbit skin to survive dehydration from the frozen state. Particular attention was given to the calculation of the water content of the skin at the completion of the drying process. Survival was judged by the growth of the epidermis in portions of treated skin transplanted onto the rabbit from which they had been removed. These investigators found that skin could not survive a state of dehydration in which the final overall water content was less than about 25%. Pretreatment of the tissue with glycerol solution did not increase the ability to withstand drying.

Buchanan and Lehman, also in 1952, reported that freeze-dried split-thickness skin grafts in the dog persist for only a short period of up to 22 days. Autografts and allografts dehydrated to within 36–41% of their original weight endured for an approximately equal length of time.

Despite the fact that several studies have indicated that grafts survive better after slow freezing, the opinion prevails that rapid freezing is more favorable to survival. This may be due in part to the work of Luyet and Gehenio (1940) showing that certain organisms and single cells that are killed by slow freezing can survive if frozen at ultrarapid rates. These authors contend that after ultrarapid freezing some tissues, especially if partially dehydrated, may be vitrified or solidified without crystal formation, thus avoiding damage to the cell.

According to Santoni-Rugiu (1962), the resurfacing of freeze-dried autografts of full-thickness rat skin is unsatisfactory and of poor quality as biologic dressing.

Assessment of Antigenicity in Freeze-Dried Allografts

In 1970, Abbott and Hembree reported that, unlike freshly excised full-thickness skin allografts, freeze-dried grafts in healthy murine recipients failed to elicit any significant inflammatory reaction, humoral antibody responses, or sensitivity in recipients as evidenced by a complete absence of heightened resistence against further grafts from the specific donor (see Chapter 7). These findings were confirmed by a subsequent experiment of Abbott and Sell (1972) in similar animals. Similar results indicating the lack of any significant immunologic reactions in the host in response to freeze-dried skin allografts were also obtained by Sell, Hyatt, and Gresham (1962) in burned patients, Yukna, Tow, Carroll, Vernino, and Bright (1977) in man, and Yukna, Turner, and Robinson (1977) in guinea pigs.

Evaluation of Freeze-Dried Skin Xenografts

Nonviable, freeze-dried skin grafts removed from bovine embryos and placed on the chorioallantois of the chick embryo are readily penetrated by the membranal blood vessels, but at a reduced rate when compared to viable and untreated skin xenografts (Converse, Ballantyne, Rogers, and Raisbeck 1958). Rogers and Converse (1958) observed in histologic sections of fresh and freeze-dried embryonic bovine skin applied to experimental defects in man that endothelial buds from the host bed had grown into the graft; they disintegrated within 10 days.

On the basis of combined gross, histologic, and angiographic examinations, Eastwood (1961) maintained that freeze-dried grafts of pigskin are firmly adherent to the host bed of rats with clear evidence of vascularization at 7–9 days and provide an effective cover for an average of 14 days, as compared to 21 days for freeze-dried allografts of rat skin. Subsequently the porcine graft disintegrates, coinciding with the appearance of patches of superficial desquamation and discoloration. However, the author did not exactly explain what he meant by "revascularization," which, strictly speaking, is the penetration of host vessels into the graft followed by two-way circulation. A question also arises as to whether he observed blood flow within the graft vasculature or penetration of host vessels.

Bromberg and co-workers (1965), working with freeze-dried split-thickness pig skin xenografts transplanted to mice, found no evidence of revascularization although these grafts remained soft with a minimal inflammatory reaction for 2 weeks. More recently, Toranto and associates (1974) were unable to distinguish vascularization of freeze-dried porcine split-thickness skin grafts transplanted to humans and rats from the invasion of the graft–host interface by granulation tissue. After transplanting freeze-dried skin xenografts from human donors to guinea pigs, Yukna, Turner, and Robinson (1977) collected sera and peritoneal macrophages from the recipient animals for serologic (ring precipitin test) and macrophage migration inhibitory factor assays. The results indicated that, while freeze-dried allografts serving as comparative controls did not evoke detectable antibody and cellular responses in the host, nearly all of the recipients bearing freeze-dried human xenografts had positive serologic and macrophage inhibition tests. From these findings it was concluded that, in contrast to a lack of or very weak antigenicity in freeze-dried allografts, freeze-dried xenografts are sufficiently antigenic—probably because they share similar antigens from different human donors—to stimulate immunologic responses and sensitivity in the host.

Summary

The findings appear to support the concept that the revascularization of frozen or freeze-dried skin grafts applied to man or animals is not entirely dependent on the viability of the original graft vasculature. As demonstrated in a study by Ballantyne et al. (1971), vascular ingrowth from the host site can occur readily provided the pattern of tissue grafts after preservation at low temperature is not unduly disorganized. However, Bromberg *et al.* (1965), working with freeze-dried split-thickness pig xenografts transplanted to mice, found no evidence of revascularization.

A question arises concerning the "revascularization" of skin grafts. It is generally accepted that a skin graft is successfully revascularized if there is a process of reformation and extension of capillaries from the host vessels into the graft, followed by reestablishment of a definitive graft vasculature with two-way circulation demonstrable by stereomicroscopy, injected dyes or contrast material, angiography, or other reliable assay procedures. A fenestrated plastic material or ordinary gauze placed over a raw surface becomes adherent by the penetration of endothelial buds (granulation tissue) into the graft but there is no circulation. When the material is removed after 14–16 days, there is bleeding from the tearing of the penetrating granulation tissue containing endothelial buds.

Chapter 7

Survival and Rejection of Second-Set
Skin Allografts

On the basis of their observations that a host develops a sensitivity directed specifically against further donations of an allograft from the first donor, Gibson and Medawar (1943) formulated the original hypothesis of acquired immunity. If a second graft from the same donor is applied, it is destroyed in an accelerated fashion, termed the "second-set phenomenon" by Medawar (1944, 1945). Whereas the primary graft of normal skin is generally rejected within 7–8 days after application, second-set grafts seldom survive beyond 5–6 days. Additional repeat-set allografts show no further shortening of the recipient's rejection time, but are destroyed at the same rate as the second-set grafts (Lehrfeld, Taylor, and Converse 1955; Rapaport and Converse 1958) (see the section on The White Graft Reaction).

Converse, Ballantyne, and Woisky (1958) have shown that a rabbit skin allograft must be in continuous contact with its host for at least 48 hours to elicit heightened resistance against further skin challenges from the specific donor. Similar results have been observed in mice by McKhann and Berrian (1959a, b) and Henry and Dammin (1962). Thus, 48 hours or more after transplantation from one donor, the host is in a "specifically sensitivity" condition against further applications of either similar or dissimilar tissues from that donor.

Acceptance and Vascularization of Repeat-Set Skin Grafts

Phase of Serum Imbibition

The experiments demonstrating the phase of serum imbibition (plasmatic circulation) have been limited to first-set skin grafts. The mechanism of serum imbibition of second-set skin grafts placed in an animal previously conditioned by a first-set graft from the same donor is not known.

Phase of Graft Revascularization

Medawar (1944) studied histologic events occurring in the second-set orthotopic skin allografts in recipient rabbits that had previously received
sensitizing primary grafts of skin from the same donor. Despite the findings
that the second-set graft is destroyed more rapidly as compared to the
first-set graft, the second-set graft survives long enough to be vascularized
by the host capillaries. At 4 days after grafting the majority of these blood
vessels are converted into "wound vessels" with a simple endothelial layer
and are obviously dilated and engorged with red corpuscles (Fig. 57). During
the period of vascularization the adhesion of the graft to its host site is often
weak, the epithelial degeneration is usually in progress, and the inflammatory reaction is precocious in its time of onset.

Vital Microscopic Studies

Using the direct skin stereomicroscopic method of evaluation, Lehrfeld,
Taylor, and Converse (1954, 1955) observed that, in rats, when second-set
allografts are transplanted up to 5 days or between 8 and 30 days after the
application of immunizing first-set grafts, they become revascularized in a

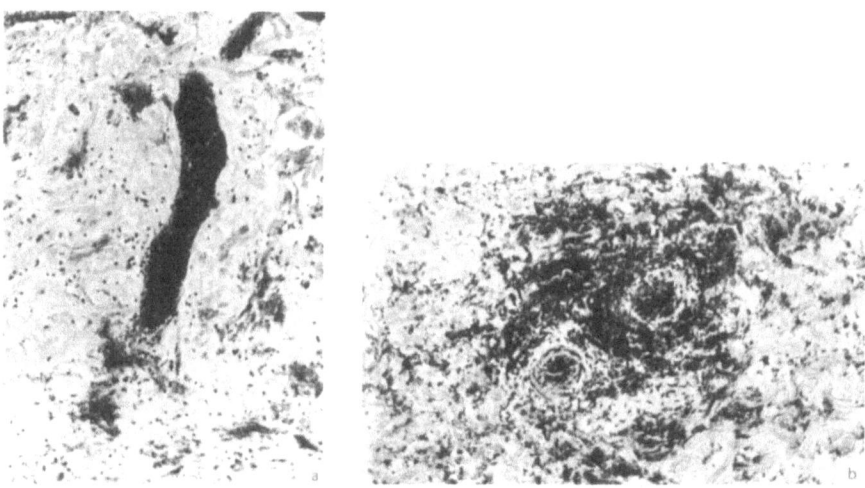

Fig. 57 a and b. Precocious breakdown of the primary vessels in a second-set
allograft 4 days after grafting. Small vessels have differentiated to form a "definitive circulation" in the lower reaches of the dermis (b). Hemorrhage is
prominent in panel b, but as panel a shows more clearly, no significant
number of native leukocytes have been able to pass through the vessel walls.
×90. Medawar (1944) J. Anat. 78:176, Cambridge University Press.

fashion similar to that of the first-set grafts. At 24 hours after transplantation there is a network of endothelial channels that are more numerous and distended than those in the normal adjacent host skin. During the next 2 days a progressive increase in the number, ramification, and dilation of the graft vasculature is observed; blood flow within the graft vascular system resumes its normal rate of velocity in at least 72 hours. In general outline, the changes occurring in the repeat-set grafts closely resemble those in the immunizing first-set, which also serve as comparative controls for that period of time; the latter changes, in turn, are similar to the stereomicroscopic findings in single-set skin grafts in adult rats reported by Taylor and Lehrfeld (1953, 1955) and by Ballantyne and Converse (1957, 1959) during the first 3 days after grafting.

Rapaport and Converse (1958) cited stereomicroscopic evidence of the successful reestablishment of a definitive vasculature with brisk blood flow in the repeat-set allografts of human skin transplanted from the same donor to the same host. In hosts who do not develop a response characteristic of a white graft reaction (see the section on the White Graft Reaction), the second-set grafts usually appear pale on the first day after transplantation, becoming pink on either the second or third day; this development is characterized by the stereomicroscopic appearance of active blood flow and filling of the graft vascular system with erythrocytes.

Histochemical Studies

The reports of Lehrfeld, Taylor, and Converse (1953, 1955) describing the vascular patterns occurring in the second-set allografts of rat skin were subsequently confirmed by Ballantyne, Platt, and Converse (1963, 1965) in similar animals by means of combined histochemical and in vivo microscopic observations. According to the stereomicroscopic findings, if the second-set skin allografts are transplanted at 4, 8, 11, and 12 days after the transplantation of first-set skin allografts from the same donor, they develop an extensive vasculature with rapid blood circulation, usually within 4–6 days. [If the interval between first-set and second-set grafts is 6 or 7 days, most of the second-set grafts undergo a white graft reaction (see the section on the White Graft Reaction).] Furthermore, using neotetrazolium and DPNH as sensitive enzyme–histochemical criteria for assessing DPN diaphorase activity in the grafted tissue, Ballantyne et al. (1965) demonstrated that at 24 hours after transplantation new capillaries originating as buds from distended vessels in the recipient site have crossed into the dermal undersurface of the second-set grafts (Fig. 58a).

By 48 hours the new endothelial channels are more numerous and have penetrated approximately one-half of the graft thickness. The parallel ingrowth of new host vessels perpendicularly toward the dermoepidermal junction of repeat-set grafts in the rat forms a characteristic pattern that

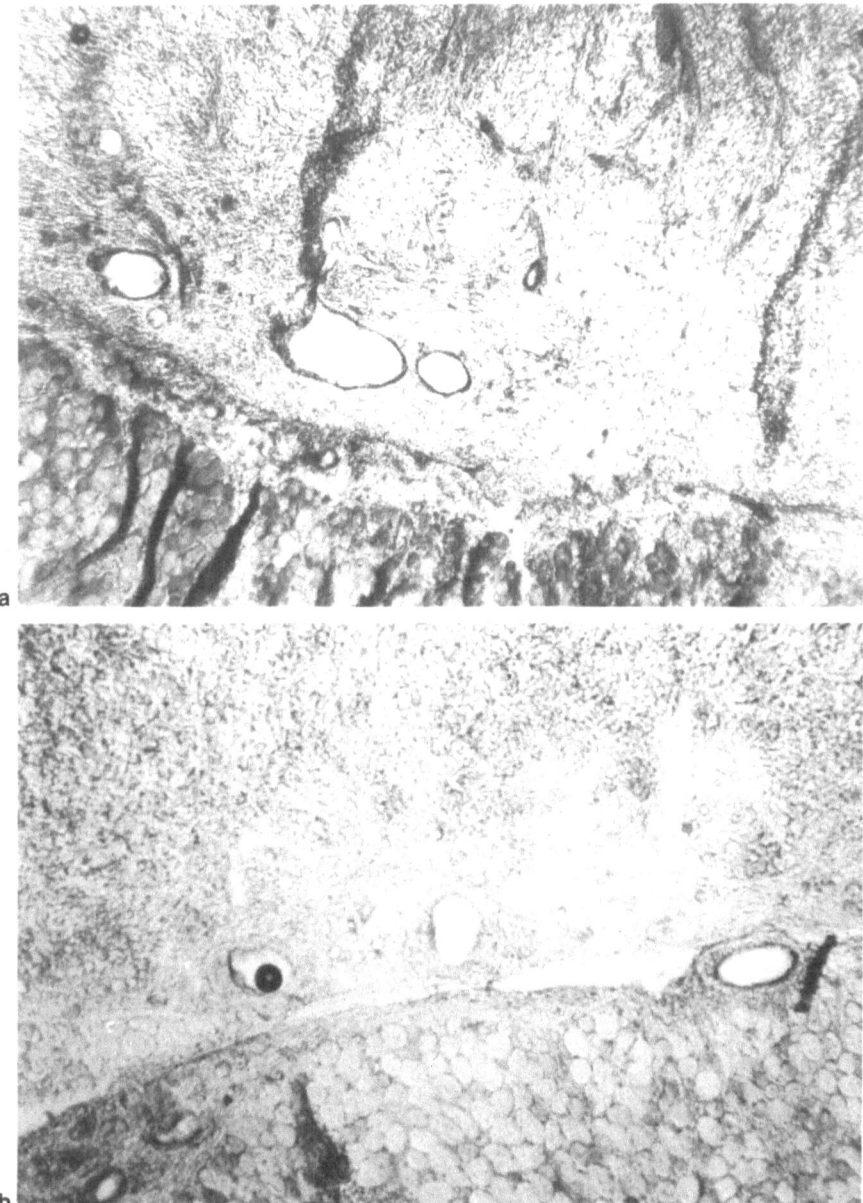

Fig. 58 a and b. Comparison of second-set allograft undergoing typical development with one undergoing a white graft reaction. ×46. **a.** Note that the typical second-set allograft at 2 days is highly vascularized and contains tissue elements with high enzymatic activity when compared to 2-day white grafts, as shown in panel b. **b.** Note the early disappearance of the enzymatic activity in the blood vessels and the tissue elements at 2 days in the allograft undergoing the white graft reaction. Ballantyne, Platt, and Converse (1965) Transplantation 3:1, © (1965) The Williams & Wilkins Co., Baltimore.

differs from the vasculature normally observed in intact adjacent host skin but is similar to the pattern seen in autografts and first-set allografts as described previously by Converse and Ballantyne (1962) in the rat. The vessels in the graft are not only more numerous but also show greater ramifications and distention than those in normal skin. In contrast, the original graft vessels indicate a progressive loss of normal enzymatic (diaphorase) activity during the first 2 days and by 3 days are difficult to discern.

Other Experimental Studies

Henry and associates (1962) reported that the histologic sequence of events in second-set human allografts closely resembles that in control autografts and in single- or first-set allografts during the first 3 days after transplantation. Vascularization accompanied by vascular distention in the repeat-set grafts commences on the second day, achieving its maximum by the fifth day. The investigators attributed the restoration of blood supply in the repeat-set grafts to the "inosculation of the patent original capillaries in the deeper dermal layers of the graft with the capillary loops from the host bed," in a fashion similar to the events occurring in control autografts and first-set allografts.

A number of experimenters (Egdahl et al. 1957; Woodruff 1960) doubted the validity of vascularization in the repeat-set skin allografts because of the greatly reduced survival time and a more violent reaction of accelerated rejection; such grafts survive temporarily, however, in a vegetative state and undergo ischemic necrosis. According to Woodruff and Simpson (1955), second-set allografts of rat split-thickness skin grafts, although they survive for the first 4–5 days, are pale, slightly swollen, rigid, and poorly adherent to the host bed; this is confirmed by the histologic appearance of capillary hemorrhages and epithelial degeneration (Fig. 33h and i). A similar observation was made by Egdahl et al. (1957) in a subsequent experiment in which second-set rabbit skin allografts were evaluated by vital microscopy and tested by intradermal injections of fluorescein. The absence of demonstrable blood circulation and failure of the fluorescein test as well as the discoloration and hardening of these grafts by the fourth to fifth day after transplantation have been offered as prima-facie evidence of the graft's failure to become vascularized.

Accelerated Rejection Phenomenon

In rabbits, as Medawar first described in 1944, repeat-set skin grafts transplanted to a recipient that has earlier received and responded to skin grafts from the same donor source become swollen and undergo a rapid transition from the shiny white of the freshly excised tissue to a dirty yellow or yellowish brown color by the fourth day. Concurrent histologic examination of the challenging tissue shows that, apart from complete suppression of epidermal cell proliferation, the invasion by leukocytes from the host is profoundly modified and appears limited to the host bed. These events are accompanied by blood stagnation and partial or total disruption of the endothelial walls of the graft blood vessels. By the eighth day the vessels have disappeared and most grafts have disintegrated. Medawar (1945, 1946), working with rabbits, and Billingham, Brent, and Medawar (1954), working with mice, have confirmed and extended these observations.

Different results have been recorded by Rolle and associates (1959), who assessed the repeat-set allografts of mouse skin by means of direct in vitro microscopic and histologic examination. They maintained that the course of changes occurring in the challenging grafts is identical to that in first-set grafts, except that the rejection begins 3–4 days earlier; furthermore, the immune reaction is identical to that seen in the first-set graft and is no more violent. This is at variance with the findings of Medawar (1944, 1945, 1946) in the rabbit and those of Billingham, Brent, and Medawar (1954) in mice that in second-set grafts the epidermal cell division is completely suppressed, the inflammatory infiltration by leukocytes is greatly modified and confined to the graft base, and the grafts survive in a "vegetative" condition.

All second-set allografts of guinea pig split-thickness skin, according to Bauer (1958), are characterized by a complete absence of primary healing and vascularization, reflected by a gross appearance of pale white color and nonadherence of the graft to its bed. In addition, none of these grafts present the characteristic features of color changes, induration, or swelling noted in the initial tissue grafts. Bauer concluded that, as applied to guinea pigs, the avascular white graft second-set reaction is a manifestation of a high level of tissue immunity, a graft rejection reaction qualitatively different from that in other animal species under similar conditions. This is at variance with a previous report by Sparrow (1953) that by 8 days after grafting most second-set skin allografts in the guinea pig are already highly swollen and are covered by thick, dark scabs.

Stereomicroscopic Studies

Lehrfeld and co-workers (1954, 1955), working with rats, found that, with the exception of the timing of the course of events, the gross and stereomicroscopic appearance of second-set grafts closely resembles that of the first-set grafts. The complete cessation of blood flow within the graft vascular system, as stressed by the authors, is one of the earliest observable indications of the onset of the immune response: the repeat-set grafts in rats immunized by skin grafts from the same donor are destroyed between 4 and

5 days after transplantation, compared to the average first-set survival time of 8 days.

A similar conclusion was reached by Ballantyne and associates (1965), who employed stereomicroscopy and histochemistry in following the course of diaphorase activity in the orthotopic second-set allografts of full-thickness rat skin. Their postoperative observations of challenging grafts just prior to and during the typical accelerated rejection reaction are in accord with the findings of Taylor and Lehrfeld (1955) and Ballantyne and Converse (1957, 1959) in similar animals in the process of rejecting single-set grafts. However, compared to the course of events observed in the first-set tissue, complete cessation of blood flow, vascular disruption, and necrotic extravasations appear earlier in the second-set skin allografts, usually 4–6 days after transplantation.

Rejection Reaction and Recall Flare in Man

Events leading to the rejection of repeat-set skin allografts after application of the preceding graft from the same donor were grossly and stereomicroscopically evaluated by Rapaport and Converse (1957, 1958) in normal human subjects. After the third day, and usually within 24 hours, all grafts were surrounded by intense erythema and edema and showed thrombosis, capillary breakdown, and hemorrhagic extravasation in rapid succession. Complete escarification of the graft was observed by the seventh day.

It was observed by Rapaport and Converse in 1957 that at the time of accelerated rejection of a subsequent skin allograft in man, a vigorous reaction of erythema and edema, termed the recall flare (Fig. 59a and b), develops at the quiescent site of the previously rejected skin allograft from the same donor. There are many well-described analogies to this phenomenon in the annals of delayed hypersensitivity. Its occurrence, for example, has been described at the site of previously negative tests in patients who had become tuberculin positive by leukocytic transfer of tuberculin hypersensitivity (H. S. Lawrence 1949).

Histologic Evaluation of Human Skin Allografts

On the basis of their histologic evaluation of successive allografts of human skin, Henry and associates (1962) stated that blood flow ceases on the fifth day after the operative procedure; this is associated with considerable vascular dilation within the donor dermis and rapid deterioration of the graft epidermis (Fig. 60a). By the end of this period the polymorphonuclear cell infiltrate in the dermis has resolved, but occasional cells may be found in the basal layer of the graft epidermis. By 8 days the rejection process is completed. It was concluded that in the accelerated phenomenon of rejection the transplantation immunity induced by the first-set allograft is

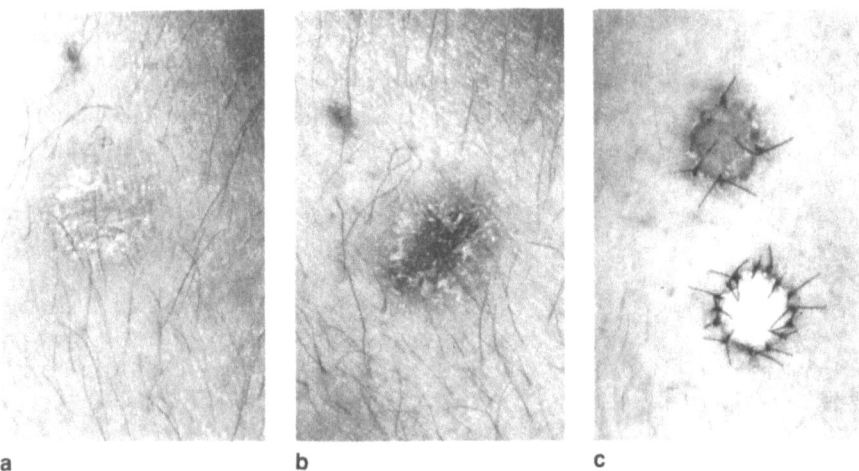

a   b   c

Fig. 59 a–c. Reactions to repeat-set skin allografts. **a.** Quiescent site of previously rejected skin allograft (repeat-set allograft No. 3). **b.** Recall flare and hemorrhagic necrosis of previously quiescent skin allograft site (repeat-set allograft No. 3) at the time of rejection of repeat-set allograft. **c.** White graft reaction in allograft 5 days after transplantation *(bottom).* Normal appearing allograft 5 days after transplantation *(top).* Rapaport and Converse (1958) Ann. Surg. 147:273.

adequate to cause an early thrombosis prior to the cellular influx, thus leading to early and rapid ischemic necrosis of the grafted tissue.

Other Experimental Studies

Working with members of various mouse strain combinations and their F_2 progeny, Eichwald, Wetzel, and Lustgraaf (1966) described the histologic appearance of second-set tail skin allografts. Depending on the method of host sensitization and the specific donor–host combinations—particularly the total number of donor antigens (determined by the degree of histocompatibility differences between donor and host)—such grafts undergo one of the three distinctive modes of a second-set reaction of accelerated rejection. In order of increasing intensity of host immune responses, the second-set grafts were classified by the authors as "blue," "red," and "white" grafts. Histologically, red grafts are characterized by vascular distention and engorgement, dermal hemorrhage, epithelial necrosis, and an absence of lymphocytic infiltration. In terms of intensity and degree, the altered reactivity resembles that seen in typical second-set allografts. In contrast, white grafts demonstrate a complete absence of vascularization coupled with a very early and rapid tissue necrosis, whereas blue grafts exhibit a well-preserved or hyperplastic epithelium and marked lymphocytic infiltration.

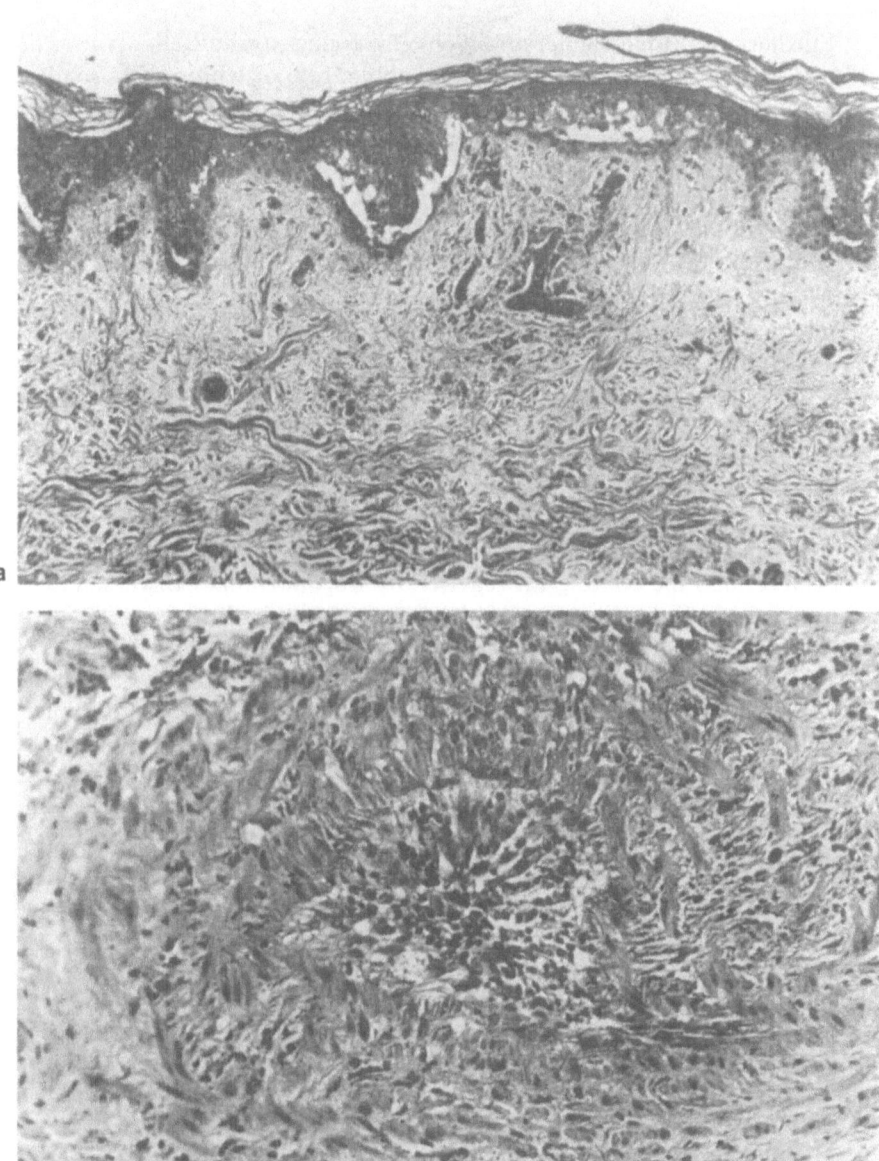

Fig. 60 a and b. Rejection reactions to repeat-set allografts of human skin. **a.** Accelerated rejection on day 4 after grafting. The superficial epidermis is dead and separating from the intact basal layer. Dilated blood vessels are present in the upper dermis. H & E. ×80. **b.** White graft reaction on day 4 after grafting. A medium-sized vein in the host tissues in the graft bed showing proliferation of the endothelial cells and infiltration of the wall with lymphocytes. The lumen is occluded but there is no evidence of thrombosis. H & E. ×168. Henry, Marshall, Friedman, Dammin, and Merrill (1962) J. Clin. Invest. 41:420.

Furthermore, Eichwald *et al.* (1966) also found, as did Ballantyne *et al.* (1965) in the rat, that instead of becoming blue, red, or white grafts some of the second-set skin grafts underwent a course of immune rejection that manifested the characteristics of both red and white grafts.

White Graft Reaction

Immune Responses

According to the report of Rapaport and Converse (1958), a peculiar form of secondary response appears when a second-set skin allograft in man is transplanted within 1 week after the rejection of the preceding allograft from the same donor. When observed by stereomicroscopy, the vascularization of such a graft is defective; grossly, the graft remains white (Fig. 59c). Their observations are in agreement with previous work by Lehrfeld, Taylor, and Converse (1954, 1955), who showed that, in rats, when the interval between first- and second-set grafting is 6 or 7 days, the second-set grafts do not develop an active blood circulation. This peculiar type of immune response has been termed the white graft reaction by Rapaport and Converse (1958) and has been confirmed in man by subsequent studies by Rapaport, Thomas, Converse, and Lawrence (1960), Henry *et al.* (1962) (Fig. 60b), Marshall *et al.* (1962), and Rapaport, Lawrence, Thomas, Converse, Tillett, and Mulholland (1962). Most investigators concluded that, in contrast to typical second-set allografts, which develop active blood circulation before the rejection time, the white graft does not become effectively vascularized and is not accepted even temporarily by its host (Lehrfeld, Taylor, and Converse 1954, 1955; Stetson 1959a, b).

The assumption that white grafts are avascular has been based on several criteria, including their failure to bleed when sliced (Stetson and Demopoluos 1958; H. S. Lawrence 1959; Stetson 1959b), their absence of observable blood circulation (Lehrfeld, Taylor, and Converse 1954, 1955; Rapaport and associates 1958, 1960, 1962), and the failure of intravenously injected dyes to enter the graft (Stetson 1959b). Each of these criteria, however, is a measure of blood circulation, rather than "revascularization," which, strictly speaking, is the process of reformation and extension of vascular capillaries.

Histologic evidence of early degeneration of the graft vessels has been cited in support of the nonvascularization of white grafts by Chutná (1961), Chutná and Polorná (1961), and Henry *et al.* (1962). However, an enzyme histochemical study of DPN diaphorase activity in white grafts of rat skin undertaken by Ballantyne and associates (1965) indicated that, while the preexisting graft vessels degenerate rapidly, new vessels originating as capillary buds from host vessels in the recipient site cross into the deep dermis of a white graft within the first 24 hours after transplantation. Then the new vessels make no further progress and rapidly degenerate (Fig. 58b). In contrast, the vascularization in typical second-set allografts continues until, by 48–72 hours, the vessels have reached the dermoepidermal junction of the graft. It would appear, therefore, that while the vasculature of the white grafts never develops sufficiently to support blood circulation, the process of revascularization is initiated just as it is in other grafts, but it is interrupted by a very early and rapid onset of immune rejection.

Although the histochemical experiment of Ballantyne *et al.* (1965) has shown that, in rats of the specific strains employed, new host capillaries invade the deep dermis of the white graft, the investigators did not imply that this process of attempted vascularization takes place in white grafts occurring in other strains of rats, in other species of animals, or in man. It is possible that the white graft reaction may vary in intensity depending on the species of animal, genetic disparity, or method of sensitization, just as the intensity of response to first-set allografts varies with these factors. For example, rejection of white grafts in animals treated with Freund's adjuvant may be so rapid as to preclude even an abortive attempt at revascularization.

Of particular interest is the unexpected observation that in some of the recipient rats bearing two skin allografts transplanted concurrently from a single donor, one graft underwent a typical accelerated rejection reaction while the other indicated a white graft reaction. However, as explained by Ballantyne *et al.* (1965), the mechanisms responsible for the appearance of two types of immune response to skin allografts from a single donor are not definitely understood. It is possible that the balance between the two patterns of immune reaction is highly delicate and also that the eventual fate of an allograft may not be entirely dependent on the level of immunity elicited in the recipient. A similar phenomenon was also observed by Eichwald *et al.* (1966) in mice following concurrent transplantation of two tail skin grafts from a single donor to the same recipient bed.

In 1970 Lambert evaluated the immune specificity of the vascular response in the acceptance and rejection of rabbit skin allografts by means of microangiography combined with autoradiographic and histologic procedures. In recipients presensitized with the specific donor cells, the grafts may either fail to become vascularized—i.e., become white grafts—or the graft vessels may lose their function soon after presumed initial vascularization. The author attributed this to an immune interaction between antibody and the homologous transplantation antigen affecting the internal environment of a graft so as to cause a functional impairment of the graft vasculature.

"Survival Time" of White Grafts

A question arises concerning the "survival time" of white grafts. It is generally held that the white graft is not accepted even temporarily by its host and that its survival time is zero (Lehrfeld, Taylor, and Converse, 1954, 1955; Stetson and Demopoulos 1958; Stetson 1959a, b). If one assumes that the cessation of blood flow represents the end point of the survival time of a graft (Taylor and Lehrfeld 1955), what then constitutes the survival time of a white graft, which never develops hemal circulation? It has been shown by Converse and Ballantyne (1962) that in rats the deterioration of new vessels in first-set skin allografts is evident histochemically before cessation of blood flow and is therefore perhaps the earliest sign of allograft rejection. According to the histochemical criterion, white grafts in rats appear to survive for at least 24 hours after transplantation. During this time period, the enzymatic activity is demonstrable in the epidermis and pilosebaceous structures of the white grafts, as well as in the new capillaries from the host. By 24–48 hours most of the enzymatic activity in the epidermis and pilosebaceous structures has disappeared and the new vessels indicate degenerative changes. In view of these findings, it has been assumed by Ballantyne and co-workers (1965) that the white graft, although not surviving long enough to allow for the establishment of blood circulation, is accepted by the host for a brief period, long enough to permit the ingrowth of a few host vessels, and that its survival time varies between 24 and 48 hours.

There is little doubt that in all the various clinical and experimental studies described thus far the observations concerning the morphologic characteristics of white grafts—with particular reference to the gross and microscopic appearance, vascular alteration, and early necrosis of the graft—are consistent and substantially correct. However, as Eichwald *et al.* (1976) have suggested, in consideration of these important findings, there is a need for further studies to elucidate the underlying mechanisms by which white grafts invariably fail to become effectively vascularized and undergo very early ischemic necrosis. A question also arises as to whether the early development of white graft ischemia is the result of a vascular failure and, if so, whether the degeneration occurs primarily in the graft or host vessels.

To resolve these questions and also to determine the association between ischemia and necrosis of the graft, Eichwald *et al.* (1976), working with white grafts of mouse tail skin, undertook a variety of different experimental procedures: (1) histology and electron microscopy of graft biopsies; (2) histologic assessment of graft viability after isogeneic retransplantation; (3) intraperitoneal injections of trypan blue; (4) intravenous injections of ^{125}I-labeled bovine serum albumin for testing radioactivity in the graft; (5) autoradiography; (6) encasing skin grafts in Millipore diffusion chambers that are subsequently positioned in the animal peritoneal cavity; (7) culture in organ culture dishes; and (8) culture in Leighton roller tubes. In all series of experiments using various combinations of different test methods, the general appearance, tissue viability, and morphologic features of white grafts were compared with those of control grafts. The controls included tail skin isografts and allografts which manifested the overt signs of an acute immune rejection reaction in normal unconditioned mouse recipients and the typical accelerated second-set phenomenon in specifically sensitized animal hosts.

Comparative evaluations of the test and control grafts placed in Millipore chambers, cultured in organ culture dishes and roller tubes, or retransplanted to syngeneic recipients provided strong experimental evidence against the interference with plasmatic circulation by the white graft reaction. Furthermore, no loss of tissue viability due to the absence of a blood supply was observed in control grafts after a 72-hour incubation in Millipore chambers, organ dishes, or roller tubes. These findings, combined with the measurements of tritiated thymidine uptake and the degree of skin discoloration after injections with trypan blue, have led Eichwald et al. (1976) to suggest that ischemia is not the actual source of early necrosis in white grafts.

Instead, as tentatively interpreted by the investigators, due to the nonthrombotic, nonnecrotizing, and obliterative changes in the original graft vasculature at the dermal undersurface of white grafts produced by a very early and rapid immune assault, the invading host vessels fail to develop anastomotic units with those of the white graft. Consequently, the entire graft turn white and becomes necrotic within 24 hours after grafting, rendering it ischemic.

In a subsequent study, Eichwald and Dolberg (1977) repeated the experimental procedure with mice for further histologic and electron microscopic evaluations and arrived at similar conclusions.

From various convincing lines of experimental evidence accumulated by Eichwald et al. (1966, 1976), Lambert (1970), and Eichwald and Dolberg (1977), the present interpretation is that white grafts survive for at least 24 hours after skin grafting, long enough to allow initial vascular proliferation in the host bed, rapidly followed by the ingrowth of host vessels into the deep dermis of the graft. Within this short period, white grafts closely resemble skin allografts placed on unconditioned recipients or typical second-set allografts transplanted to recipients that have been previously immunized by similar or dissimilar tissues from a specific donor. However, because the very early and ultrarapid onset of the immune response causes early degenerative changes in the original graft vessels and extensive tissue necrosis of the graft, white grafts are unable to preserve their viability long enough for the invading host vessels to establish an adequate blood circulation within the graft dermis and/or to develop functional vascular anastomoses with the original graft vasculature. These interpretations are in line with those of Ballantyne et al. (1965).

However, despite additional information describing the nature, behavior, and structural changes of white grafts, the question of the survival time of these grafts remains unresolved.

Chronic Rejection Patterns of Second-Set Grafts

Until 1958, the rejection of second-set repeat-set allografts had been considered by most investigators to be a classically consistent and acute phenomenon. However, in 1960, Rogers and associates, working with noninbred rats, showed that a certain percentage of second- and third-set reactions are significantly different when the donor and host are closely related to each other in certain donor–host combinations. In second- and third-set reciprocal skin interchanges between closely related rats a certain proportion of grafts were characterized by typical acute second- and third-set reactions, a certain percentage by subacute second- and third-set reactions, a smaller percentage by chronic second-set reactions, and an even smaller percentage by prolonged survival second-set reactions.

Similar observations on variations of the second-set phenomenon have also been described by Peer, Walia, and Pullen (1960) in skin grafts exchanged between human parents and their young offspring and by Hildemann and Walford (1960) in the Syrian hamster. The variations in the second- and third-set responses have been separated into three categories and defined by Hildemann and Walford (1960); they are termed *rapid chronic rejections, intermediate chronic rejections,* and *prolonged chronic rejections.*

The course of events associated with these variations in the second- and third-set responses closely resembles that observed in first-set grafts undergoing an analogous type of chronic rejection.

Behavior and Fate of Second-Set Massive Allografts

Evidence was accumulated by Ballantyne, Siegel, and Converse (1963) that second-set massive grafts of allogeneic skin fail to be destroyed in an accelerated fashion in recipient rats that have previously received either small or massive skin grafts from the same donor. In contrast, control small second-set allografts in a similarly conditioned host undergo a typical accelerated rejection reaction.

Gross and stereomicroscopic observations in situ of the challenging massive grafts resemble those of first-set grafts of similar dosage and are in accord with the findings of Converse, Siegel, and Ballantyne (1962, 1963) in single-set massive grafts in similar animals. At 3 or 4 days after transplantation, there is active blood flow in the vasculature of the second-set grafts and an initial decline in the vessel dilation is noted during the firs few days. Thereafter, until just prior to the onset of the rejection response, the graft blood vessels progressively resume the pattern of vessels in normal intact skin.

The slowing and eventual cessation of blood flow coinciding with the distention of blood vessels and followed by vascular disruption are early stereomicroscopic indications of impending tissue breakdown. Some of the grafts with prolonged survival undergo a slow chronic rejection similar to that described by Hildemann and Walford (1960) in the Syrian hamster and referred to as "melting away" by Converse, Siegel, and Ballantyne (1962,

1963). This melting away reaction consists of a series of small hemorrhages with subsequent undermining in several places along the graft margins and occurs cyclically, giving the transplant an appearance of being nibbed, similar to that observed in first-set massive allografts (see the section on Other Experimental Studies in Chapter 5).

Summary

The accelerated rejection of second-set skin allografts in recipients that had previously received transplants of similar or dissimilar tissues from the same or a specific donor is a well-known phenomenon in transplantation immunity. This phenomenon has been extensively investigated in various species systems. Most previous clinical and experimental studies using challenging orthotopic skin grafts as a transplantation model were primarily designed to determine (1) the genetic loci of histocompatibility antigens, (2) the degree and type of histocompatibility difference between individuals, (3) the nature of immune responsiveness in the host, (4) the interaction between the humoral and cellular reactions, or (5) the efficiency of immunosuppressive agents. However, unlike reports on single- or first-set skin grafts, there are comparatively few reports that describe the course of the histopathologic changes that take place in second-set skin allografts placed on specifically sensitized recipients.

Since the first detailed report by Medawar in 1944, ample evidence accumulated from subsequent clinical and research studies (Lehrfeld, Taylor, and Converse 1954, 1955; Rapaport and Converse 1958; Rolle et al. 1959; Henry et al. 1962; Ballantyne et al. 1965) shows that second-set orthotopic skin grafts, if not undergoing a white graft rejection reaction, survive long enough to receive a direct blood supply from the recipient. However, the mode of vascularization in second-set allografts, as that in first sets, remains a subject of considerable discussion.

On the other hand, a few investigators (Woodruff and Simpson 1955; Egdahl et al. 1957; Bauer 1958; Woodruff 1960) were unable to demonstrate evidence of vascularization in such grafts.

References

Abbott, W. M., Hembree, J. S. (1970). Absence of antigenicity in freeze-dried skin allografts. Cryobiology 6:416.

Abbott, W. M., Sell, K. W. (1972). Alteration of histocompatibility and species antigens in skin by freeze-drying. Surg. Forum 23:282.

Adams, R. A., Patt, D. I., Lutz, B. R. (1956). Long term persistence of skin homografts in untreated hamsters. Transplant. Bull. 3:41.

Algire, G. H. (1943a). An adaptation of the transparent-chamber technique to the mouse. J. Natl. Cancer Inst. 4:1.

Algire, G. H. (1943b). Microscopic studies of the early growth of a transplantable melanoma of the mouse, using the transparent-chamber technique. J. Natl. Cancer Inst. 4:13.

Algire, G. H., Legallais, F. Y. (1949). Recent developments in the transparent-chamber technique as adapted to the mouse. J. Natl. Cancer Inst. 10:225.

Allgöwer, M., Blocker, T. G., Jr. (1952). Viability of skin in relation to various methods of storage. Tex. Rep. Biol. Med. 10:3.

Anderson, D., Billingham, R. E., Lampkin, G. H., Medawar, P. B. (1951). The use of skin grafting to distinguish between monozygotic and dizygotic twins in cattle. Heredity 5:379.

Antopol, W., Glaubach, S., Goldman, L. (1950). The use of neotetrazolium as a tool in the study of active cell processes. Trans. N.Y. Acad. Sci. 12:156.

Arguedas, J. M., Pérez-Tamayo, R. (1958). The pattern of wound healing of skin autografts and skin homografts in the rat. Surg. Gynecol. Obstet. 106:671.

Artz, C. P., Rittenbury, M. S., Yarbrough, D. R., III (1972). An appraisal of allografts and xenografts as biological dressings for wounds and burns. Ann. Surg. 175:934.

Avery, G. B., Hunt, C. V. (1966). The use of supravital staining to evaluate the survival of skin homografts. Transplantation 4:755.

Bach, F. H., Amos, D. B. (1967). Hu-1: Major histocompatibility locus in man. Science 156:1506.

Bailey, B. N., Lewis, S. R., Blocker, T. G., Jr. (1962). Influence of thermal trauma *per se* on homograft survival: An experimental study. Tex. Rep. Biol. Med. 20:30.

Ballantyne, D. L., Jr. (1960). Discussion of: Hildemann, W. H., Walford, R. L. Chronic skin homograft rejection in the Syrian hamster. Ann. N.Y. Acad. Sci. 87:71.

Ballantyne, D. L., Jr., Cascarano, J., Converse, J. M. (1964). Histochemical diagnosis of homograft rejection. Ann. N.Y. Acad. Sci. 120:46.

Ballantyne, D. L., Jr., Converse, J. M. (1957). The relation of hair cycles to the survival time of suprapannicular and subpannicular skin homografts in rats. Ann. N.Y. Acad. Sci. 64:958.

Ballantyne, D. L., Jr., Converse, J. M. (1958). Vascularization of composite auricular grafts transplanted to the chorio-allantois of the chick embryo. Transplant. Bull. 5:373.

Ballantyne, D. L., Jr., Converse, J. M. (1959). Further observations of hair-skin cycles and the survival of skin homografts in rats. Transplant. Bull. 6:93.

Ballantyne, D. L., Jr., Converse, J. M. (1966). Structure and properties of skin and of its components from the point of view of preservation by freezing and freeze-drying. Cryobiology 3:131.

Ballantyne, D. L., Jr., Hawthorne, G. A., Rees, T. D., Seidman, I. (1971). An experimental evaluation of skin graft preservation with silicone fluid. Cryobiology 8:211.

Ballantyne, D. L., Jr., Platt, J. M., Converse, J. M. (1963). Comparative study of the vascularization of white graft and typical second-set skin homografts in the rat. Surg. Forum 14:472.

Ballantyne, D. L., Jr., Platt, J. M., Converse, J. M. (1965). Vascularization of second-set homografts in the rat, with particular reference to the white graft: A histochemical study. Transplantation 3:1.

Ballantyne, D. L., Jr., Siegel, W. H., Converse, J. M. (1963). The behavior of massive skin homografts in adoptively and actively immunized rats. Plast. Reconstr. Surg. 32:310.

Ballantyne, D. L., Jr., Siegel, W. H., Kapitchnikov, M. M. (1962). Further observations on massive skin homografts in rats. Transplant. Bull. 30:143.

Ballantyne, D. L., Jr., Stetson, C. A., Jr. (1964). Serologic reactions to skin homografts of various sizes in the rat. Ann. N.Y. Acad. Sci. 120:7.

Ballantyne, D. L., Jr., Uhlschmid, G. K., Converse, J. M. (1969). Massive rabbit skin xenografts in rats. Transplantation 7:274.

Barker, C. F., Billingham, R. E. (1967). The role of regional lymphatics in the skin homograft response. Transplantation 5:962.

Barker, C. F., Billingham, R. E. (1968). The role of afferent lymphatics in the rejection of skin homografts. J. Exp. Med. 128:197.

Barlyn, L. W., Berggren, R. B., Lehr, H. B. (1944). Frozen skin autografts protected by dimethyl sulfoxide. Surg. Forum 15:475.

Barnes, A. D., Krohn, P. L. (1957). The estimation of the number of histocompatibility genes controlling the successful transplantation of normal skin in mice. Proc. R. Soc. Lond. [Biol.] 146:505.

Baronio, G. (1804). Degli Innesti Animali. Stamperia e Fonderia del Genio, Milano.

Batchelor, J. R., Hackett, M. (1970). HL-A matching in treatment of burned patients with skin allografts. Lancet 2:581.

Bauer, J. A., Jr. (1958). Histocompatibility in inbred strains of guinea pigs. Ann. N.Y. Acad. Sci. 73:663.

Bellman, S., Velander, E. (1957). Vascular reaction following experimental transplantation of free full thickness skin grafts. In: Transactions of the International Society of Plastic Surgeons, First Congress, Stockholm and Uppsala, 1955. Williams & Wilkins, Baltimore, p. 493.

Bellman, S., Velander, E., Frank, H. A., Lambert, P. B. (1964). Survival of arteries in experimental full-thickness skin autografts. Transplantation 2:167.

Ben-Hur, N. (1974). Commentary on: Toranto, I. R., Salyer, K. E., Myers, M. B. Vascularization of porcine skin heterografts. Plast. Reconstr. Surg. 54:352.

Ben-Hur, N., Solowey, A. C., Rapaport, F. T. (1969a). The xenograft rejection phenomenon. I. Response of the mouse to rabbit, guinea pig and rat skin xenografts. Isr. J. Med. Sci. 5:1.

Ben-Hur, N., Solowey, A. C., Rapaport, F. T. (1969b). The xenograft rejection phenomenon. II. Response of the guinea pig to mouse, rat and rabbit skin xenografts. Isr. J. Med. Sci. 5:322.

Berggren, R. B., Lehr, H. B. (1965). Clinical use of viable frozen human skin. J.A.M.A. 194:129.

Berrian, J. H., McKhann, C. F. (1960). Transplantation immunity involving the H-3 locus: Graft survival times. J. Natl. Cancer Inst. 25:111.

Bert, P. (1865). Expériences de greffe animale. C. R. Soc. Biol. [4] (Paris) 1:172.

Billingham, R. E. (1959). Reactions of grafts against their hosts. Science 130:947.

Billingham, R. E. (1961). Free skin grafting in mammals. In: Billingham, R. E., Silvers, W. K. (eds.) Transplantation of Tissues and Cells. Wistar Institute Press, Philadelphia, Chapter 1, pp. 1–24.

Billingham, R. E., Barker, C. F. (1969). Recent developments in transplantation immunology, Part I. Plast. Reconstr. Surg. 43:559.

Billingham, R. E., Boswell, T. (1953). Studies on the problem of corneal homografts. Proc. R. Soc., Lond. [Biol.] 141:392.

Billingham, R. E., Brent, L., Medawar, P. B. (1953). 'Actively acquired tolerance' of foreign cells. Nature 172:603.

Billingham, R. E., Brent, L., Medawar, P. B. (1954). Quantitative studies on tissue transplantation immunity. II. The origin, strength and duration of actively and adoptively acquired immunity. Proc. R. Soc., Lond. [Biol.] 143:58.

Billingham, R. E., Brent, L., Medawar, P. B., Sparrow, E. M. (1954). Quantitative studies on tissue transplantation immunity. I. The survival times of skin homografts exchanged between members of different inbred strains of mice. Proc. R. Soc., Lond. [Biol.] 143:43.

Billingham, R. E., Hildemann, W. H. (1958a). Studies of transplantation immunity in hamsters. Ann. N.Y. Acad. Sci. 73:676.

Billingham, R. E., Hildemann, W. H. (1958b). Studies on the immunological responses of hamsters to skin homografts. Proc. R. Soc., Lond. [Biol.] 148:216.

Billingham, R. E., Hodge, B. A., Silvers, W. K. (1962). An estimate of the number of histocompatibility loci in the rat. Proc. Natl. Acad. Sci. U.S.A. 48:138.

Billingham, R. E., Krohn, P. L., Medawar, P. B. (1951). Effect of cortisone on survival of skin homografts in rabbits. Brit. Med. J., 1:1157.

Billingham, R. E., Lampkin, G. H., Medawar, P. B., Williams, H. L. (1952). Tolerance to homografts, twin diagnosis, and the freemartin condition in cattle. Heredity 6:201.

Billingham, R. E., Medawar, P. B. (1951). The technique of free skin grafting in mammals. J. Exp. Biol. 28:385.

Billingham, R. E., Medawar, P. B. (1952). The freezing, drying and storage of mammalian skin. Brt. J. Exp. Biol. 29:454.

Billingham, R. E., Sawchuck, G. H., Silvers, W. K. (1960). Studies on the histocompatibility genes of the Syrian hamster. Proc. Natl. Acad. Sci. U.S.A. 46:1079.

Billingham, R. E., Silvers, W. K. (1959). Inbred animals and tissue transplantation immunity. Transplant. Bull. 6:399.

Billingham, R. E., Silvers, W. K. (1962). Studies on cheek pouch skin homografts in the Syrian hamster. In: Wolstenholme, G. E. W., Cameron, M. P. (eds.) Ciba Foundation Symposium on Transplantation. Little, Brown, Boston, pp. 90–108.

Billingham, R., Silvers, W. K. (1971). The Immunobiology of Transplantation. Prentice-Hall, Englewood Cliffs, N.J.

Birch, J., Brånemark, P.-I. (1969). The vascularization of a free full thickness skin graft. I. A vital microscopic study. Scand. J. Plast. Reconstr. Surg. 3:1.

Birch, J., Brånemark, P.-I., Lundskog, J. (1969). The vascularization of a free full thickness skin graft. II. A microangiographic study. Scand. J. Plast. Reconstr. Surg. 3:11.

Birch, J., Brånemark, P.-I., Nilsson, K. (1969). The vascularization of a free full thickness skin graft. III. An infrared thermographic study. Scand. J. Plast. Reconstr. Surg. 3:18.

Blandford, S. E., Garcia, F. A. (1953). Case report: Successful homogenous skin graft in a severe burn using an identical twin as donor. Plast. Reconstr. Surg. 11:31.

Blank, H., Coriell, L. L., Scott, T. F. M. (1948). Human skin grafted upon the chorioallantois of the chick embryo for virus cultivation. Proc. Soc. Exp. Biol. Med. 69:341.

Bondoc, C. C., Burke, J. F. (1971). Clinical experience with viable frozen human skin and a frozen skin bank. Ann. Surg. 174:371.

Brånemark, P.-I., Lindström, J. (1963). A modified rabbit's ear chamber. High-power, high-resolution studies in regenerated and preformed tissues. Anat. Rec. 145:553.

Braun, W. (1899). Klinisch-histologische Untersuchungen über die Anheilung ungestielter Hautlappen. Beitr. Klin. Chir. 25:211.

Breedis, C., Barnes, W. A., Furth, J. (1937). Effect of rate of freezing on the transmitting agent of neoplasms of mice. Proc. Soc. Exp. Biol. Med. 36:220.

Brent, L. (1958). Tissue transplantation immunity. Prog. Allergy 5:271.

Briggs, R., Jund, L. (1944). Successful grafting of frozen and thawed mouse skin. Anat. Rec. 89:75.

Bromberg, B. E., Song, I. C. (1966). Skin substitutes, homo-, and heterografts. Am. J. Surg. 112:28.

Bromberg, B. E., Song, I. C., Mohn, M. P. (1965). The use of pig skin as a temporary biological dressing. Plast. Reconstr. Surg. 36:80.

Brown, J. B. (1937). Homografting of skin: With report of success in identical twins. Surgery 1:558.

Brown, J. B., Fryer, M. P., Randall, P., Lu, M. (1953). Postmortem homografts as "biological dressings" for extensive burns and denuded areas. Immediate and preserved homografts as life-saving procedures. Ann. Surg. 138:618.

Buchanan, F. T., Lehman, E. P. (1952). An experimental study of preservation of skin grafts by the freeze-drying process. Surg. Forum 2:637.

Burleson, R., Eisman, B. (1972). Nature of the bond between partial-thickness skin and wound granulations. Surgery 72:315.

Burleson, R., Eisman, B. (1973). Mechanisms of antibacterial effect of biologic dressings. Ann. Surg. 177:181.

Burns Unit, First Affiliated Hospital of Hou, Number 2 Unit. Chinese People's Liberation Army (1973). A review of the management of extensive third degree burns in 14 successive years. Chin. Med. J., No. 11 (Nov.), p. 148.

Butcher, E. O. (1934). The hair cycles in the albino rats. Anat. Rec. 61:5.

Calnan, J., Kulatilake, A. W. (1962). Small versus massive skin homograft survival in the rat. Br. J. Plast. Surg. 15:341.

Carrel, A. (1912). The preservation of tissues and its application in surgery. J.A.M.A. 59:523.

Casson, P., Solowey, A. C., Converse, J. M., Rapaport, F. T. (1966). Delayed hypersensitivity status of burned patients. Surg. Forum 17:268.

Castermans, A. (1957). Vascularization of skin grafts. Transplant. Bull. 4:153.

Ceppellini, R., Curtoni, E. S., Mattiuz, P. L., Leigheb, G., Visetti, M., Colombi, A. (1966). Survival of test skin grafts in man: Effect of genetic relationship and of blood groups incompatibility. Ann. N.Y. Acad. Sci. 129:421.

Chai, C. K. (1974). Genetic studies of histocompatibility in rabbits: Identification of major and minor genes. Immunogenetics 1:126.

Chambers, R., Hale, H. P. (1932). The formation of ice in protoplasm. Proc. R. Soc., Lond. [Biol.] 110:336.

Chutná, J. (1961). White-graft reaction and passive transfer of immunity in inbred strains of mice. Transplant. Bull. 28:23.

Chutná, J., Pokorná, Z. (1961). Study of the local reaction in immunized hosts under conditions leading to "white grafts" and notes on the question of the mechanism of action of humoral antibodies on skin homografts. Folia Biol. (Praha) 7:32.

Clemmesen, Th. (1962). The early circulation in split skin grafts. Acta Chir. Scand. 124:11.

Clemmesen, Th. (1964). The early circulation in split-skin grafts. Restoration of blood supply to split-skin autografts. Acta Chir. Scand. 127:1.

Clemmesen, Th. (1967). Experimental studies on the healing of free skin autografts. Dan. Med. Bull., 14 [Suppl. II]: p. 1.

Cohen, N. (1971). Amphibian transplantation reactions: A review. Am. Zool. 11:193.

Colson, P., Leclerq, P., Gangolphe, M., Houot, R., Janvier, H., Prunieras, M. (1959). Utilisation des homogreffes alternées avec des autogreffes dans le traitement des grand brules. II. Étude histo-biologique. Ann. Chir. Plast 4:177.

Converse, J. M., Ballantyne, D. L., Jr. (1962). Distribution of diphosphopyridine nucleotide diaphorase in rat skin autografts and homografts. Plast. Reconstr. Surg. 30:415.

Converse, J. M., Ballantyne, D. L., Jr., Rogers, B. O., Raisbeck, A. P. (1957). "Plasmatic circulation" in skin grafts. Transplant. Bull. 4:154.

Converse, J. M., Ballantyne, D. L., Jr., Rogers, B. O., Raisbeck, A. P. (1958). A study of viable and non-viable skin grafts transplanted to the chorio-allantoic membrane of the chick embryo. Transplant. Bull. 5:108.

Converse, J. M., Ballantyne, D. L., Jr., Woisky, J. (1958). The vascularization of skin homografts and transplantation immunity. Ann. N.Y. Acad. Sci. 73:693.

Converse, J. M., Duchet, G. (1947). Successful homologous skin grafting in a war burn using an identical twin as donor. Plast. Reconstr. Surg. 2:342.

Converse, J. M., Filler, M., Ballantyne, D. L., Jr. (1965). Vascularization of split-thickness skin autografts in the rat. Transplantation 3:22.

Converse, J. M., McCarthy, J. G., Brauer, R. O., Ballantyne, D. L., Jr. (1977). Transplantation of skin: Grafts and flaps. In: Converse, J. M. (ed.) Reconstructive Plastic Surgery, Vol. 1. Saunders, Philadelphia, Chapter 6, pp. 152–239.

Converse, J. M., Rapaport, F. T. (1956). The vascularization of skin autografts and homografts: An experimental study in man. Ann. Surg. 143:306.

Converse, J. M., Rapaport, F. T. (1957). Observations on experimental skin homografts in man. In: Transactions of the International Society of Plastic Surgeons, First Congress, Stockholm and Uppsala, 1955. Williams & Wilkins, Baltimore, p. 473.

Converse, J. M., Siegel, W. H., Ballantyne, D. L., Jr. (1962). Studies in antigenic overloading with massive skin homografts in rats. In: Mechanisms of Immunological Tolerance. Hašek, M., Lengerová, A., and Vijtisková, M. (eds.), Proceedings of a Symposium, at Liblice, Czechoslovakia. Publishing House of the Czechoslovak Academy of Sciences, Prague, pp. 277–283.

Converse, J. M., Siegel, W. H., Ballantyne, D. L., Jr. (1963). Studies in antigenic overloading with massive skin homografts in rats. Plast. Reconstr. Surg. 31:9.

Converse, J. M., Šmahel, J., Ballantyne, D. L., Jr., Harper, A. D. (1975). Inosculation of vessels of skin graft and host bed: A fortuitous encounter. Br. J. Plast. Surg. 28:274.

Converse, J. M., Uhlschmid, G. K., Ballantyne, D. L., Jr. (1969). "Plasmatic circulation" in skin grafts. The phase of serum imbibition. Plast. Reconstr. Surg. 43:495.

Conway, H., Griffith, B. H., Shannon, J. E., Jr., Findley, A. (1957). Re-examination of the transparent chamber technique as applied to the study of circulation in autografts and homografts of the skin. Plast. Reconstr. Surg. 20:103.

Conway, H., Joslin, D., Rees, T. D., Stark, R. B. (1952). Observations on the development of circulation in skin grafts. III. Morphologic changes observed in homologous skin grafts. Plast. Reconstr. Surg. 9:557.

Conway, H., Joslin, D., Stark, R. B. (1951). Observations on the development of circulation in skin grafts. I. Technique of adaptation of the transparent chamber technique to study of the circulation in skin grafts. Plast. Reconstr. Surg. 8:194.

Conway, H., Sedar, J. D., Shannon, J. E., Jr. (1957). Re-evaluation of the transparent chamber technique in the study of the circulation in autografts and homografts of skin. Transplant. Bull. 4:62.

Conway, H., Stark, R. B., Joslin, D. (1951). Observations on the development of circulation in skin grafts. II. The physiologic pattern of early circulation in auto-grafts. Plast. Reconstr. Surg. 8:312.

Counce, S., Smith, P. Barth, R., Snell, G. D. (1956). Strong and weak histocompatibility gene differences in mice and their role in the rejection of homografts of tumors and skin. Ann. Surg. 144:198.

Dammin, G. J., Couch, N. P., Murray, J. E. (1957). Prolonged survival of skin homografts in uremic patients. Ann. N.Y. Acad. Sci. 64:967.

Dammin, G. J., Murray, J. E. (1959). Criteria for acceptance of skin grafts. Transplant, Bull. 6:429.

Daniller, A. I., Ballantyne, D. L., Jr., Converse, J. M. (1971). Prolonged skin allograft survival achieved by in vivo cooling. Transplant. Proc. 3:860.

Davis, J. S., Traut, H. F. (1925). Origin and development of the blood supply of whole-thickness skin grafts. An experimental study. Ann. Surg. 82:871.

De Stefano, C. (1959). Ricerche sull'attivita' enzimatica di lembi di cute in trapianti omologhi. Boll. Soc. Ital. Biol. Sper. 35:1719.

Donaldson, R. C., Payne, J., Hershey, F. B. (1960). Effects of storage on enzyme activity and viability of skin. Surg. Gynecol. Obstet. 110:419.

Douglas, B. (1944). The treatment of burns and other extensive wounds with special emphasis on the transparent jacket system. Surgery 15:96.

Duncan, W. R., Streilein, J. W. (1978a). Analysis of the major histocompatibility complex in Syrian hamsters. I. Skin graft rejection, graft-versus-host reactions, mixed lymphocyte reactions, and immune response genes in inbred strains. Transplantation 25:12.

Duncan, W. R., Streilein, J. W. (1978b). Analysis of the major histocompatibility complex in Syrian hamsters. II. Linkage studies. Transplantation 25:17.

Eade, G. G. (1958). The relationship between granulation tissue, bacteria, and skin grafts in burned patients. Plast. Reconstr. Surg. 22:42.

Eastwood, D. S. (1961). Observations on skin heterografts in rats. Br. J. Plast. Surg. 14:160.

Edgerton, M. T., Edgerton, P. J. (1955). Vascularization of homografts. Transplant. Bull. 2:98.

Edgerton, M. T., Peterson, H. A., Edgerton, P. J. (1957). The homograft rejection mechanism. Arch. Surg. 74:238.

Egdahl, R. H., Good, R. A., Varco, R. L. (1957). Studies in homograft and heterograft survival. Surgery 42:228.

Egdahl, R. H., Varco, R. L. (1956). Intradermal fluorescein test for homograft rejection period. Transplant. Bull. 3:152.

Egdahl, R. H., Varco, R. L., Good, R. A. (1958). Local reactions and lymph node response to skin heterografts between rabbits and rats. Int. Arch. Allergy Appl. Immunol. 13:129.

Eichwald, E. J., Dolberg, M. (1977). Hyperacute rejection of murine skin grafts. Transplantation 23:516.

Eichwald, E. J., Pay, G., Busath, D., Smith, C. (1976). Ischemic versus cytotoxic damage in the white graft reaction. Transplantation 22:86.

Eichwald, E. J., Silmser, C. R. (1955). Communication. Transplant. Bull. 2:148.

Eichwald, E. J., Silmser, C. R., Wheeler, N. (1957). The genetics of skin grafting. Ann. N.Y. Acad. Sci. 64:737.

Eichwald, E. J., Wetzel, B., Lustgraaf, E. C. (1966). Genetic aspects of second-set skin grafts in mice. Transplantation 4:260.

Elliott, R. A., Jr., Hoehn, J. G. (1973). Use of commercial porcine skin for wound dressings. Plast. Reconstr. Surg. 52:401.

Enderlen (1897). Histologische Untersuchungen über die Einheilung von Propfungen nach Thiersch and Krause. Dtsch. Z. Chir. 45:453.

Etheredge, E. E., Shons, A., Harris, N., Najarian, J. S. (1971). Prolongation of skin xenograft survival by L-asparaginase. Transplantation 11:353.

Feller, I., DeWeese, M. S. (1958). The use of stored cutaneous autografts in wound treatment. Surgery 44:540.

Flatt, A. E. (1948). Refrigerated autogenous skin grafting. A review of 50 cases. Lancet 2:249.

Franklin, R. M., Prendergast, R. A. (1970). Primary rejection of skin allografts in the anterior chamber of the rabbit eye. J. Immunol. 104:463.

Gabb, B. W. Piazza, A., d'Amaro, J., Balner, H. (1972). Genetics of RhL-A system of rhesus monkeys. Transplant. Proc. 4:11.

Gardner, R. J., Preston, F. W. (1962). Prolonged skin homograft survival in advanced cancer and cirrhosis of the liver. Surg. Gynecol. Obstet. 115:399.

Garré, C. (1889). Über die histologischen Vorgänge bei der Anheilung der Thiersch' schen. Transplantionen. Beitr. Klin. Chir. 4:625.

Georgiade, N., Peschel, E., Georgiade, R., Brown, I. (1956). A clinical and experimental investigation of the preservation of skin. Plast. Reconstr. Surg. 17:267.

Gibson, T., Medawar, P. B. (1943). The fate of skin homografts in man. J. Anat. 77:299.

Goldmann, E. E. (1890). Die künstliche Ueberhäutung offener Krebse durch Hauttransplantationen nach Thiersch. Zentralbl. Allg. Pathol. 1:505.

Goodpasture, E. W., Douglas, B., Anderson, K. (1938). A study of human skin grafted upon the chorio-allantois of chick embryos. J. Exp. Med. 68:891.

Gorer, P. A. (1938). The antigenic basis of tumor transplantation. J. Pathol. Bacteriol. 47:231.

Gorer, P. A. (1942). The role of antibodies in immunity to transplanted leukaemia in mice. J. Pathol. Bacteriol. 54:51.

Gorer, P. A. (1960). Transplantese. Ann. N.Y. Acad. Sci. 87:604.

Gorer, P. A., Loutit, J. F., Micklem, H. S. (1961). Proposed revision of 'transplantese.' Nature 189:1024.

Gotjamanos, T. (1970). The effect of skin allograft size on survival time following transplantation between mice differing at the H-2 locus. Aust. J. Exp. Biol. Med. Sci. 48:1.

Graham, J. B., Petersons, N. (1965). Skin homografts in patients with cancer of the cervix. Can. Med. Assoc. J. 92:60.

Green, H., Lorincz, A. L. (1956). Growth of mouse tumor in the chick embryo with retention of capacity by the chick to form antibody cells to the tumor in later life. Nature 178:146.

Green, I., Corso, P. F. (1959). A study of skin homografting in patients with lymphomas. Blood 14:235.

Greene, H. S. N. (1955). Compatibility and noncompatibility. Ann. N.Y. Acad. Sci. 59:311.

Gresham, R. B., Perry, V. P., Thompson, V. K. (1963). Practical methods of short-term storage of homografts. Arch. Surg. 87:417.

Gruber, R. P., Kaplan, E. N., Lucas, Z. J. (1974). Skin homografts in rats compared to other organ transplantations. Plast. Reconstr. Surg. 53:64.

Guthy, E. A., Billote, J. B., Burke, J. F. (1974). Skin as an organ transplant. A critical re-evaluation of the allografts. Chir. Plast. (Berl.) 2:263.

Hall, J. G. (1967). Studies of the cells in the afferent and efferent lymph of lymph nodes draining the site of skin homografts. J. Exp. Med. 125:737.

Haller, J. A., Jr., Billingham, R. E. (1964). Preliminary studies on the origin of the vasculature in free skin grafts. In: Montagna, W., Billingham, R. E. (eds.) Advances in Biology of Skin, Vol. 5, Wound Healing. MacMillan, New York, Chapter 10, p. 165.

Haller, J. A., Jr., Billingham, R. E. (1967). Studies of the origin of the vasculature in free skin grafts. Ann. Surg. 166:896.

Haller, J. A., Jr., Rauenhorst, J., Adkins, J., Billingham, R. E. (1966). Origin of the vasculature in skin grafts. Surg. Forum 17:96.

Ham, A. W. (1952). Some histophysiological problems peculiar to calcified tissues. J. Bone Joint Surg. [Am.] 34:701.

Hanks, J. H., Wallace, R. E. (1949). Relation of oxygen and temperature in the preservation of tissues by refrigeration. Proc. Soc. Exp. Biol. Med. 71:196.

Harris, N. S., Abston, S. (1974). Antiporcine antibodies in xenografted burned patients. J. Surg. Res. 16:599.

Henle, A. (1899). Klinische und experimentelle Beiträge zur Lehre von der transplantation ungestielter Hautlappen. II. Experimenteller Teil. Beitr. Klin. Chir. 24:615.

Henry, L., Dammin, G. J. (1962). Time and dose relationships in the development of immunity to skin homografts in mice. J. Immunol. 89:841.

Henry, L., Marshall, D. C., Friedman, E. A., Dammin, G. J., Merrill, J. P. (1962). The rejection of skin homografts in the normal human subject. Part II. Histological findings. J. Clin. Invest. 41:420.

Henry, L., Marshall, D. C., Friedman, E. A., Goldstein, D. P., Dammin, G. J. (1961). A histologic study of the human skin autograft. Am. J. Pathol. 39:317.

Hildemann, W. H. (1957). Scale homotransplantation in goldfish. (Carassius auratus). Ann. N.Y. Acad. Sci. 64:775.

Hildemann, W. H., Haas, R. (1960). Comparative studies of homotransplantation in fishes. J. Cell. Comp. Physiol. 55:227.

Hildemann, W. H., Walford, R. L. (1960). Chronic skin homograft rejection in the Syrian hamster. Ann. N.Y. Acad. Sci. 87:56.

Hoerr, N. L. (1936). Cytological studies by the Altmann-Gersh freezing-drying method. I. Recent advances in the technique. Anat. Rec. 65:293.

Hübscher, C. (1888). Beiträge zue Hautverpflanzung nach Thiersch. Beitr. Klin. Chir. 4:395.

Hyatt, G. W., Turner, T. C., Bassett, C. A. L., Pate, J. W., Sawyer, P. N. (1952). New methods for preserving bone, skin and blood vessels. Postgrad. Med. 12:239.

Hynes, W. (1954). The early circulation in skin grafts with a consideration of methods to encourage their survival. Br. J. Plast. Surg. 6:257.

Jackson, D. (1954). A clinical study of the use of skin homografts for burns. Br. J. Plast. Surg. 7:26.

Jasani, M. K., Lewis, G. P. (1971). Lymph flow and changes in intracellular enzymes during healing and rejection of rabbit skin grafts. J. Physiol. 219:525.

Jensen, C. O. (1903). Experimentelle Untersuchungen über Krebs bei Mäusen. Zentralbl. Bakteriol. [Naturwiss.] 34:28.

Joslin, D. (1952). Tissue chamber and splint for the mouse. Science 115:601.

Jungengel, M. (1891). Die Hauttransplantation nach Thiersch. Verh. Phys. Med. Ges. Würzb. 25:1.

Kamrin, B. B. (1960). Studies on the healing of successful homografts in albino rats. Ann. N.Y. Acad. Sci. 87:323.

Kamrin, B. B. (1961). Analysis of the union between host and graft in the albino rat. Plast. Reconstr. Surg. 28:221.

Kapitchnikov, M. M., Ballantyne, D. L., Jr., Setson, C. A. (1962). Immunological reactions to skin homotransplantation in rabbits and rats. Ann. N.Y. Acad. Sci. 99:497.

Kaplan, H. J., Stevens, T. R. (1975). A reconsideration of immunological privilege within the anterior chamber of the eye. Transplantation 19:302.

Keeley, R. L. A., Gomez, A. C., Brown, I. W., Jr. (1952). An experimental study of the effects of freezing, partial dehydration, and ultra-rapid cooling on the survival of dog skin grafts. Plast. Reconstr. Surg. 9:330.

Kikuchi, I., Omori, M. (1970). Demonstration of leaking vessels under skin grafts. Plast. Reconstr. Surg. 45:66.

Kiyono, K., Sueyasu, Y. (1917). The experimental study in avian embryo after inoculation of tissues from various animals. I. Further classification of species for inoculation. Kyoto Igaku Zassi 14:68.

Kohayakawa, K. (1966). Determination of skin homograft survival endpoints by Disulphine Blue. Med. J. Osaka Univ. 16:425.

Kountz, S. L., Williams, M. A., Williams, P. L., Kapros, C., Dempster, W. J. (1963). Mechanism of rejection of homotransplanted kidneys. Nature 199:257.

Kubáček, V. (1962). Significance of the epidermal layer of the skin for the take of a free skin graft. Acta Chir. Plast. 4:197.

Lambert, P. B. (1970). The effect of immunity on the vascularization of skin allografts. Transplantation 10:463.

Lambert, P. B., Frank, H. A. (1967). Local recognition of histocompatibility differences in skin grafts. Science 155:99.

Lapp, W. S., Bliss, J. Q. (1966). Skin graft size: Its effect on graft survival in mice incompatible at a weak locus. Transplantation 4:754.

Lappé, M. A., Graff, R. G., Snell, G. D. (1969). The importance of target size in the destruction of skin grafts with non-H-2 incompatibility. Transplantation 7:372.

Law, E. J., Nathan, P., MacMillan, B. G. (1970). Clinical experience with porcine xenografts. In: Matter, P., Barclay, T. L., Konickova, Z. (eds.) Research in Burns, Transactions of the Third International Congress on Research in Burns, Prague. Huber, Bern, p. 281.

Lawrence, H. S. (1949). The cellular transfer of cutaneous hypersensitivity to tuberculin in man. Proc. Soc. Exp. Biol. Med. 71:516.

Lawrence, H. S. (1959). Homograft sensitivity—An expression of the immunologic origins and consequences of individuality. Physiol. Rev. 39:811.

Lawrence, J. C. (1972). Storage and skin metabolism. Br. J. Plast. Surg. 25:440.

Lehr, H. B., Berggren, R. B., Lotke, P. A., Coriell, L. L. (1964). Permanent survival of preserved skin autografts. Surgery 56:742.

Lehrfeld, J. W., Taylor, A. C. (1953). The dosage phenomenon in rat skin homografts. Plast. Reconstr. Surg. 12:432.

Lehrfeld, J. W., Taylor, A. C., Converse, J. M. (1954). Relation of survival time to implantation time of second set skin homografts in the rat. Proc. Soc. Exp. Biol. Med. 86:849.

Lehrfeld, J. W., Taylor, A. C., Converse, J. M. (1955). Observations on second and third set skin homografts in the rat. Plast. Reconstr. Surg. 15:74.

Leight, G. S., Kirkman, R., Rasmusen, B. A., Rosenberg, S. A., Sachs, D. H., Terrill, R., Melville, G. (1978). Transplantation in miniature swine. III. Effects of MSLA and A-O blood group matching on skin allograft survival. Tissue Antigens 12:65.

Leight, G. S., Sachs, D. H., Rosenberg, S. A. (1977). Transplantation in miniature swine. II. In vitro parameters of histocompatibility in MSLA homozygous mini pigs. Transplantation 23:271.

Lewis, T. (1927). The Blood Vessels of the Human Skin and Their Responses. Shaw & Sons, London.

Ljungqvist, A., Almgård, L. A. (1966). The vascular reaction in the free skin allo- and autografts. A stereomicro-angiographic and histological study in the rabbit. Acta Pathol. Microbiol. Scand. 68:553.

Loeb, L. (1945). The Biological Basis of Individuality. Thomas, Springfield, Ill.

Loeb, L., Addison, W. H. F. (1909). Beiträge zur Analyse des Gewebewachstums. 2. Transplantation der Haut des Meeschweinchens in Tiere verschiedener Spezies. Arch Entwickl. Organ. 27:73.

Loeb, L., Addison, W. H. F. (1911). Beiträge zur Analyse des Gewebewachstums. V. Ueber die Transplantation der Taubenhaut in die Taube und in andere Tierarten. Arch. Entwickl. Organ. 32:44.

Lombard, W. P. (1911–1912). The blood pressure in the arterioles, capillaries, and small veins of the human skin. Am. J. Physiol. 29:335.

Lovelock, J. E. (1953). The hemolysis of human red blood cells by freezing and thawing. Biochem. Biophys. Acta 10:414.

Lovelock, J. E. (1954). Biophysical aspects of the freezing and thawing of living cells. Proc. R. Soc. Med. 47:60.

Luyet, B. J., Gehenio, P. M. (1940). Life and death at low temperatures. Diodynamics (Monograph on General Physiology, No. 1), Normandy, Mo.

Marckmann, A. (1965a). Autologous skin grafts in the rat. Uptake of ^{35}S-sulfate. Proc. Soc. Exp. Biol. Med. 119:557.

Marckmann, A. (1965b). Autologous skin grafts in the rat. Biochemical analysis of mucopolysaccharides and hydroxyproline. Proc. Soc. Exp. Biol. Med. 119:794.

Marckmann, A. (1966). Autologous skin grafts in the rat: Vital microscopic studies of the microcirculation. Angiology 17:475.

Marckmann, A. (1967). Biology of skin autografts. Dan. Med. Bull. 14:135.

Marckmann, A., Zachariae, H. (1964). Histamine in full-thickness skin autografts of rat. Proc. Soc. Exp. Biol. Med. 117:705.

Markley, K., Thornton, S. W. (1973). Skin graft prolongation caused by changes in grafting procedure. Transplantation 16:80.

Markley, K., Thornton, S. W., Smallman, E. (1971). The effect of traumatic and nontraumatic shock on allograft survival. Surgery 70:667.

Marrangoni, A. G. (1950). An experimental study on refrigerated skin grafts stored in ten per cent homologous serum. Plast. Reconstr. Surg. 6:425.

Marshall, D. C., Friedman, E. A., Goldstein, D. P., Henry, L., Merrill, J. P. (1962). The rejection of skin homografts in the normal human subject. Part I. Clinical observations. J. Clin. Invest. 41:411.

Matter, P., Chambler, K., Lewis, S. R., Blocker, T. G., Jr. (1963). Relationship between survival time and size of homografts in rats. Transplantation 1:157.

Matthews, D. N. (1945). Storage of skin for autogenous grafts. Lancet 1:775.

McCabe, W. P., Rebuck, J. W., Kelly, A. P., Jr., Ditmars, D. M., Jr. (1973). Cellular immune response of humans to pigskin. Plast. Reconstr. Surg. 51:181.

McDonald, J. C. (1968). Rejection of skin allografts by healthy humans. Relationship of type of rejection to degree of immunity. Arch. Surg. 97:306.

McGregor, I. A. (1955a). The vascularization of human skin. Br. J. Plast. Surg. 7:331.

McGregor, I. A. (1955b). Vascularization of homografts of human skin. Transplant. Bull. 2:11.

McKhann, C. F. (1964). Transplantation studies of strong and weak histocompatibility barriers in mice. I. Immunization. Transplantation 2:613.

McKhann, C. F., Berrian, J. H. (1959a). Transplantation immunity: Some properties of induction and expression. Ann. Surg. 150:1025.

McKhann, C. F., Berrian, J. H. (1959b). Time relationships in the induction of transplantation immunity. Transplant. Bull. 6:428.

McKhann, C. F., Berrian, J. H. (1961). Immunologic properties of weak histocompatibility genes. J. Immunol. 86:170.

McLaughlin, C. R. (1954). Composite ear grafts and their blood supply. Br. J. Plast. Surg. 7:274.

Medawar, P. B. (1944). The behavior and fate of skin autografts and skin homografts in rabbits. J. Anat. 78:176.

Medawar, P. B. (1945). A second study of behavior and fate of skin homografts in rabbits. J. Anat. 79:157.

Medawar, P. B. (1946). Immunity to homologous grafted skin. I. The suppression of cell division in grafts transplanted to immunized animals. Br. J. Exp. Pathol. 27:9.

Medawar, P. B. (1948). Immunity to homologous grafted skin. III. The fate of skin homografts transplanted to the brain, to subcutaneous tissue, and to the anterior chamber of the eye. Br. J. Exp. Pathol. 29:58.

Medawar, P. B. (1954). The storage of living skin. Proc. R. Soc. Med. 47:62.

Medawar, P. B. (1958). The immunology of transplantation. In: The Harvey Lectures, 1956–1957, Series 52. Academic Press, New York, p. 144.

Medawar, P. B. (1962). Opening remarks. In: Wolstenholme, G. E. W., Cameron, M. P. (eds.) Ciba Foundation Symposium on Transplantation. Little, Brown, Boston, p. 1.

Merwin, R. M., Algire, G. H. (1956). The role of graft and host vessels in the vascularization of grafts of normal and neoplastic tissue. J. Natl. Cancer Inst. 17:23.

Mider, G. B., Morton, J. J. (1939). The effect of freezing in vitro on some transplantable mammalian tumors and on normal rat skin. Am. J. Cancer 35:502.

Miller, T. A. (1974). The deleterious effect of split skin homograft coverage on split-skin donor sites. Plast. Reconstr. Surg. 53:316.

Miller, T. A., Switzer, W. E., Foley, F. D., Moncrief, J. A. (1967). Early homografting of second degree burns. Plast. Reconstr. Surg. 40:117.

Miller, T. A., White, W. I. (1972). Healing of second degree burns. Comparison of effects of early application of homografts and coverage with tape. Plast. Reconstr. Surg. 49:552.

Mir y Mir, L. (1951). Biology of the skin graft. New aspects to consider in its revascularization. Plast. Reconstr. Surg. 8:378.

Moore, T. C., Schayer, R. W. (1969). Histidine decarboxylase activity of autografted and allografted rat skin. Transplantation 7:99.

Mowlem, R. (1952). Skin homografts. Med. Illustrated 6:552.

Munster, A. M., Eurenius, K., Katz, R. M., Canales, L., Foley, F. D., Mortensen, R. F. (1973). Cell-mediated immunity after thermal injury. Ann. Surg. 177:139.

Murphy, J. B. (1912). Transplantability of malignant tumors to the embryos of a foreign species. J.A.M.A. 59:874.

Murphy, J. B. (1913). Transplantability of tissues to the embryo of foreign species. Its bearing on questions of tissue specificity and tumor immunity. J. Exp. Med. 17:482.

Murphy, J. B. (1914a). Studies in tissue specificity. II. The ultimate fate of mammalian tissue implanted in the chick embryo. J. Exp. Med. 19:181.

Murphy, J. B. (1914b). Factors of resistance to heteroplastic tissue-grafting. Studies in tissue specificity. III. J. Exp. Med. 19:513.

Nilsson, N., Obel, N., Schantz, B. (1971). Light permeability of skin allografts as an indicator of the homograft rejection process in the dog. Acta Chir. Scand. 137:315.

Ninnemann, J. L., Fisher, J. C., Frank, H. A. (1978). Prolonged survival of human skin allografts following thermal injury. Transplantation 25:69.

O'Donoghue, M. N., Zarem, H. A. (1971). Stimulation of neovascularization—Comparative efficacy of fresh and preserved skin grafts. Plast. Reconstr. Surg. 48:474.

Ohmori, S., Kurata, K. (1960). Experimental studies on the blood supply to various types of skin grafts in rabbits using isotope P^{32}. Plast. Reconstr. Surg. 25:547.

Owen, R. D. (1945). Immunogenetic consequences of vascular anastomoses between bovine twins. Science 102:400.

Padgett, E. C. (1932). Is iso-grafting practicable? South. Med. J. 25:895.

Padgett, E. C. (1939). Calibrated intermediate skin grafts. Surg. Gynecol. Obstet. 69:779.

Pandya, N. J., Zarem, H. A. (1974). The absence of vascularization in porcine skin grafts on mice. Plast. Reconstr. Surg. 53:211.

Pate, J. W. (1954). Transplantation of preserved non-viable tissues. In: Ciba Foundation Symposium on Preservation and Transplantation of Normal Tissues. Little, Brown, Boston, p. 60.

Pederson, F. B., Matthiessen, M. E., Garbarsch, C. (1970). Enzyme histochemical studies on rat skin autografts. Scand. J. Plast. Reconstr. Surg. 4:83.

Peer, L. A. (1956). Long survival time of skin graft from mother to male child. With biopsy section of skin graft taken 20 days after transplantation. Plast. Reconstr. Surg. 18:169.

Peer, L. A. (1957). Behavior of skin grafts interchanged between parents and infants. Transplant. Bull. 4:109.

Peer, L. A. (1958). Behavior of skin grafts exchanged between parents and offspring. Ann. N.Y. Acad. Sci. 73:584.

Peer, L. A., Bernhard, W., Walker, J. C., Jr. (1958). Full-thickness skin exchanges between parents and their children. Am. J. Surg. 95:239.

Peer, L. A., Walia, I. S., Pullen, R. (1960). Observations on partial tolerance to skin homografts in man. Transplant. Bull. 26:115.

Peer, L. A., Walker, J. C. (1951). The behavior of autogenous human tissue grafts. II. Plast. Reconstr. Surg. 7:73.

Pepper, F. J. (1954). Studies on the viability of mammalian skin autografts after storage at different temperatures. Br. J. Plast. Surg. 6:250.

Perry, V. P. (1966). A review of skin preservation. Cryobiology 3:109.

Perry, V. P., Evans, V. J., Young, J. M., Earle, W. R., Hyatt, G. W. (1957). Some recent studies with tissue culture as related to tissue transplantation. Transplant. Bull. 4:28.

Pfeffer, A. Z., Rogers, B. O. (1955). The possible role of blood group antigens in the behavior of skin homografts. A. Preliminary report. Plast. Reconstr. Surg. 15:495.

Pihl, B., Weiber, A. (1963). Studies of the vascularization of free full-thickness skin grafts with radioisotope techniques. Acta Chir. Scand. 125:19.

Polge, C., Smith, A. U., Parkes, A. S. (1949). Revival of spermatozoa after vitrification and dehydration at low temperatures. Nature 164:666.

Psillakis, J. M., de Jorge, F. B., Villardo, R., Albano, A. de M., Martins, M., Spina, V. (1969). Water and electrolyte changes in autogenous skin grafts. Discussion of the so-called "plasmatic circulation." Plast. Reconstr. Surg. 43:500.

Raju, S., Grogan, J. B. (1969a). Allograft implants in the anterior chamber of the eye of the rabbit: Early vascularization and sensitization of the host. Transplantation 7:475.

Raju, S., Grogan, J. B. (1969b). Effect of storage on skin allograft survival. Arch. Surg. 99:100.

Raju, S., Vessella, R. I., Grogan, J. B., Conn, J. H. (1974). The unreliability of visual inspection to monitor skin graft survival times in AG-B incompatible rat strains. Transplantation 17:325.

Rapaport, F. T., Converse, J. M. (1957). Observations on immunological manifestations of the homograft rejection phenomenon in man: The recall flare. N.Y. Acad. Sci. 64:836.

Rapaport, F. T., Converse, J. M. (1958). The immune response to multiple-set skin homografts. An experimental study in man. Ann. Surg. 147:273.

Rapaport, F. T., Converse, J. M., Horn, L., Ballantyne, D. L., Jr., Mulholland, J. H. (1964). Altered reactivity to skin homografts in severe thermal injury. Ann. Surg. 159:390.

Rapaport, F. T., Lawrence, H. S., Thomas, L., Converse, J. M., Tillett, W. S., Mulholland, J. H. (1962). Cross-reactions to skin homografts in man. J. Clin. Invest. 41:2166.

Rapaport, F. T., Thomas, L., Converse, J. M., Lawrence, H. S. (1960). The specificity of skin homograft rejection in man. Ann. N.Y. Acad. Sci. 87:217.

Rappaport, I., Pepino, A. T., Dietrick, W. (1970). Early use of xenografts as a biologic dressing in burn trauma. Am. J. Surg. 120:144.

Rees, T. D., Ballantyne, D. L., Jr., Hawthorne, G. A., Nathan, A. (1968). Effects of silastic sheet implants under simultaneous skin autografts in rats. Plast. Reconstr. Surg. 42:339.

Réverdin, J. L. (1872). De la greffe épidermique. Arch. Gen. Med. 19:276.

Ribbert-Göttingen, H. (1904). Ueber Transplantation auf Individuen anderer Gattung. Verh. Dtsch. Pathol. Ges. 8:104.

Rogers, B. O. (1951). Guide and bibliography for research into the skin homograft problem. Plast. Reconstr. Surg. 7:169.

Rogers, B. O. (1957a). The use of skin homografts to differentiate between monozygotic and dizygotic human twins. In: Transactions of the International Society of Plastic Surgeons, First Congress, Stockholm and Uppsala, 1955. Williams & Wilkins, Baltimore, p. 480.

Rogers, B. O. (1957b). The genetics of skin homotransplantation in the human. Ann. N.Y. Acad. Sci. 64:741.

Rogers, B. O. (1959). Transplantation of skin. In: Peer, L. A. (ed.) Transplantation of Tissues, Vol. 2. Williams & Wilkins, Baltimore, p. 73.

Rogers, B. O. (1963). Genetics of transplantation in humans. Dis. Nerv. Syst. Monogr. [Suppl.] 24:3.

Rogers, B. O., Bach, F. H. (1964). Genetics as applied to tissue homotransplantation. In: Converse, J. M. (ed.) Reconstructive Plastic Surgery. Saunders, Philadelphia, 5:2146.

Rogers, B. O., Converse, J. M. (1958). Bovine embryo skin zoografts as temporary biologic dressings for burns and other skin defects. Plast. Reconstr. Surg. 22:471.

Rogers, B. O., Converse, J. M., Silvetti, A. N. (1957). Preliminary clinical studies on bovine embryo skin grafts. Transplant. Bull. 4:24.

Rogers, B. O., Raisbeck, A. P., Ballantyne, D. L., Jr., Converse, J. M. (1960). The genetics of skin homografting in rats between brothers, sisters, parents and grandparents. In: Transactions of the International Society of Plastic Surgeons, Second Congress, London, 1959. Livingstone, Edinburgh, p. 421.

Rolle, G. K., Taylor, A. C., Charipper, H. A. (1959). A study of vascular changes in skin grafts in mice and their relationship to homograft breakdown. J. Cell. Comp. Physiol. 53:215.

Rother, K., Rother, U., Ballantyne, D. L., Jr. (1967). Serum complement activity in rat recipients of small and massive skin allografts. Proc. Soc. Exp. Biol. Med. 124:439.

Russell, P. S., Monaco, A. P. (1965). The Biology of Tissue Transplantation. Little, Brown, Boston.

Russell, P. S., Winn, H. J. (1970). Medical Progress: Transplantation. N. Engl. J. Med. 282:786, 848, 896.

Sachs, D. H., Leight, G., Cone, J., Schwarz, S., Stuart, L., Rosenberg, S. A. (1976). Transplantation in miniature swine. I. Fixation of the major histocompatibility complex. Transplantation 22:559.

Salisbury, R. E., Wilmore, D. W., Silverstein, P., Pruitt, B. A., Jr. (1973). Biologic dressings for skin graft donor sites. Arch. Surg. 106:705.

Sandison, J. C. (1924). A new method for the microscopic study of living growing tissues by the introduction of a transparent chamber in the rabbit's ear. Anat. Rec. 28:281.

Santoni-Rugiu, P. (1962). Compared studies on the viability of skin stored by different methods. Plast. Reconstr. Surg. 30:586.

Scothorne, R. J., McGregor, I. A. (1953). The vascularization of autografts and homografts of rabbit skin. J. Anat. 87:379.

Scothorne, R. J., Scothorne, A. W. (1953). Histochemical studies on human skin autografts. J. Anat. 87:22.

Scothorne, R. J., Tough, J. S. (1952). Histochemical studies of human skin autografts and homografts. Br. J. Plast. Surg. 5:161.

Sell, K. W., Hyatt, G. W., Gresham, R. B. (1962). The status of the freeze-dried skin homograft in the severely burned patient. In: Artz, C. P. (ed.) Research in Burns. Washington, D. C., and Davis, Philadelphia, pp. 351–356.

Shepard, G. H. (1972). The storage of split-skin grafts on their donor sites. Clinical and experimental study. Plast. Reconstr. Surg. 49:115.

Sherman, J. K. (1965). Pretreatment with protective substances as a factor in freeze-thaw survival. Cryobiology 1:298.

Silverstein, P , Munster, A. K., Curreri, P. W., Pruitt, B. A. (1971). The graft–host relationship of split-thickness porcine xenografts to human and animal wounds. Presented at the Third Annual Meeting of the American Burn Association, San Antonio, Texas, April.

Silvetti, A. N., Cotton, C., Bryne, R. J., Berrian, J. H., Menendez, A. F. (1957). Preliminary experimental studies of bovine embryo skin grafts. Transplant. Bull. 4:25.

Singh, S. B., Tevethia, S. S. (1973). Demonstration of mixed lymphocyte interaction in hamsters. Proc. Soc. Exp. Biol. Med. 142:443.

Šmahel, J. (1962). Revascularization of a free skin autograft. Acta Chir. Plast. 4:102.

Šmahel, J. (1967). The revascularization of a free skin autograft. Acta Chir. Plast. 9:76.

Šmahel, J. (1971a). Biology of the stage of plasmatic imbibition. Br. J. Plast. Surg. 24:140.

Šmahel, J. (1971b). Free skin transplantation on a prepared bed. Br. J. Plast. Surg. 24:129.

Šmahel, J. (1977). The healing of skin grafts. Clin. Plast. Surg. 4:409.

Šmahel, J., Bartos, F. (1967). Contribution to the problems of weight and physicochemical changes in skin autotransplants following implantation. Acta. Chir. Plast. 9:140.

Šmahel, J., Clodius, L. (1971). The blood vessel system of free human skin grafts. Plast. Reconstr. Surg. 47:61.

Šmahel, J., Ganzoni, N. (1970). Contribution to the origin of the vasculature in free skin autografts. Br. J. Plast. Surg. 23:322.

Smith, A. U. (1954). Effects of low temperatures on living cells and tissues. In: Harris, R. J. C. (ed.) Biological Applications of Freezing and Drying. Academic Press, New York, Chapter 1, p. 2.

Smith, J. W., Ringland, J., Wilson, R. (1964). Vascularization of skin grafts. Surg. Forum 15:473.

Snell, G. D. (1948). Methods for the study of histocompatibility genes. J. Genet. 49:87.

Snell, G. D. (1953). The genetics of transplantation. J. Natl. Cancer Inst. 14:691.

Snell, G. D. (1957). The homograft reaction. Ann. Rev. Microbiol. 11:439.

Snell, G. D. (1958). Histocompatibility genes of the mouse. II. Production and analysis of isogenic resistant lines. J. Natl. Cancer Inst. 21:843.

Snell, G. D. (1964). The terminology of tissue transplantation. Transplantation 2:655.

Snell, G. D. (1971). The histocompatibility systems. Transplant. Proc. 3:1133.

Snell, G. D., Cloudman, A. M. (1943). The effect of rate of freezing on the survival of fourteen transplantable tumors of mice. Cancer Res. 3:396.

Snell, G. D., Stevens, L. C. (1961). Histocompatibility genes of mice. III. H-1 and H-2, two histocompatibility loci in the first linkage group. Immunology 4:366.

Snyderman, R. K., Miller, D. G., Lizardo, J. G. (1960). Prolonged skin homograft and heterograft survival in patients with neoplastic disease. Plast. Reconstr. Surg. 26:373.

Sokolic, I. H., Farpour, A., Ulin, A. W., Howard, J. (1959). The use of heterograft skin as a biological dressing. Surg. Forum 10:847.

Song, I. C., Bromberg, B. E., Mohn, M. P., Koehnlein, E. (1966). Heterografts as biological dressing for large skin wounds. Surgery 59:576.

Sparrow, E. M. (1953). The behaviour of skin autografts and skin homografts in the guinea-pig, with special reference to the effect of cortisone acetate and ascorbic acid on the homograft reaction. J. Endocrinol. 9:101.

State, D., Peter, M. E. (1974). Clinical use of porcine xenografts in conditions other than burns. Surg. Gynecol. Obstet. 138:13.

Stetson, C. A., Jr. (1959a). The role of antibody in the rejection of homografts. In: Shaffer, J. H., LoGrippo, G. A., Chase, M. W. (eds.) Mechanisms of Hypersensitivity. Little, Brown, pp. 569–573.

Stetson, C. A., Jr. (1959b). Passive transfer of homograft immunity with serum. In: Grabar, P., Miescher, P. (eds.) Immunopathology, First International Symposium. Benno Schwabe, Basel, pp. 184–190.

Stetson, C. A. (1963). The role of humoral antibody in the homograft reaction. Adv. Immunol. 3:97.

Stetson, C. A., Jr., Demopoulos, R. (1958). Reactions of skin homografts with specific immune sera. Ann. N.Y. Acad. Sci. 73:687.

Stevens, S. M. B. (1975). The restoration of the vasculature of skin autografts in the rabbit. Pathology 7:79.

Strauch, B., Murray, D. E. (1967). Transfer of composite graft with immediate suture anastomosis of its vascular pedicle measuring less than 1 mm in external diameter using microsurgical techniques. Plast. Reconstr. Surg. 40:325.

Streilein, J. W., Billingham, R. E. (1970a). An analysis of graft-versus-host disease in Syrian hamsters. I. The epidermolytic syndrome: Description and studies on its procurement. J. Exp. Med. 132:163.

Streilein, J. W., Billingham, R. E. (1970b). An analysis of graft-versus-host disease in Syrian hamsters. II. The epidermolytic syndrome: Studies on its pathogenesis. J. Exp. Med. 132:181.

Strumia, M. M., Hodge, C. C. (1945). Frozen human skin grafts. Ann. Surg. 121:860.

Subba Rao, D. S. V., Grogan, J. B. (1977). Orthotopic skin graft survival in rats that have harbored skin implants in the anterior chamber of the eye. Transplantation 24:377.

Sugarbaker, P. H., Sabath, L. D., Morgan, A. P. (1974). Neomycin toxicity from porcine skin xenografts. Ann. Surg. 179:183.

Switzer, W. E., Moncrief, J. A., Mills, W., Jr., Order, S. E., Lindberg, R. B. (1966). The use of canine heterografts in the therapy of thermal injury. J. Trauma 6:391.

Taylor, A. C., Gerstner, R. (1956). Tissue survival after exposure to low temperatures and the effectiveness of protective pretreatments. I. Evaluation by growth in tissue culture. J. Cell. Comp. Physiol. 46:477.

Taylor, A. C., Gerstner, R., Converse, J. M. (1956). Preservation of skin grafts by refrigeration for reconstructive surgery. Plast. Reconstr. Surg. 18:275.

Taylor, A. C., Lehrfeld, J. W. (1953). Determination of survival time of skin homografts in the rat by observations of vascular changes in the graft. Plast. Reconstr. Surg. 12:423.

Taylor, A. C., Lehrfeld, J. W. (1955). Definition of survival time of homografts. Ann. N.Y. Acad. Sci. 59:351.

Teich-Alasia, S., Masera, N., Massaioli, N., Massé, C. (1961). The Disulphine Blue coloration in the study of humoral exchanges in skin grafts. Br. J. Plast. Surg. 14:308.

Terasaki, P. I., McClelland, J. D. (1964). Microdroplet assay of human serum cytotoxins. Nature 204:998.

Thiersch, C. (1874). Ueber die feineren anatomischen Veränderungen bei Aufheilung von Haut auf Granulationen. Arch. Klin. Chir. 17:318.

Thompson, N. (1962). The role of succinic dehydrogenase and sulfhydryl groups during epidermal rejection in skin homografts. A preliminary histochemical study in rats. Transplant. Bull. 30:113.

Tilney, N. L., Gowans, J. L. (1971). The sensitization of rats by allografts transplanted to alymphatic pedicles of skin. J. Exp. Med. 133:951.

Tissot, R. G., Cohen, C. (1972). Histocompatibility in the rabbit. Identification of the major locus. Tissue Antigens 2:267.

Toranto, I. R., Salyer, K. E., Myers, M. B. (1974). Vascularization of porcine skin heterografts. Plast. Reconstr. Surg. 54:195.

Vaino, U., Alfthan, O. (1969). Leucineaminopeptidase reaction and skin transplantation. Ann. Med. Exp. Fenn. 48:1.

Vanni, G. (1950). Auto and homotransplantation of skin preserved at low temperature. Plast. Reconstr. Surg. 6:161.

Veith, F. J., Murray, J. E., Miller, M. C. (1966). Massive skin grafts in dogs under immunosuppressive chemotherapy. Surgery 59:594.

Waksman, B. H. (1963). The pattern of rejection in rat skin homografts and its relation to the vascular network. Lab. Invest. 12:46.

Walker, B. E., Goldman, A. S. (1963). Thymidine-H³ radioautography of skin grafts in mice. Tex. Rep. Biol. Med. 21:425.

Wandall, J. H. (1972). Healing of split skin autografts after storage in deuterated medium. Scand. J. Plast. Reconstr. Surg. 6:36.

Ward, F. E., Mendell, N. R., Seigler, H. F., MacQueen, J. M., Amos, D. B. (1978). Factors which have a significant effect on the survival of human skin grafts. Transplantation 26:194.

Warden, G. L., Reemtsma, K., Steinmuller, D. (1973). The phenomenon of adaptation: Graft or host? Transplant. Proc. 5:635.

Webster, J. P. (1944). Refrigerated skin grafts. Ann. Surg. 120:431.

Wentscher, J. (1903). Ein weiterer Beitrag zur überlebensfähigkeit der menschlichen epidermiszellen. Dtsch. Z. Chir. 70:21.

White, E., Hildemann, W. H. (1968). Allografts in genetically defined rats: Difference in survival between kidney and skin. Science 162:1293.

Wiener, J., Pearl, J. S., Lattes, R. G., Spiro, D. (1969). Endothelial cell–leukocyte bridges in skin allografts. Transplantation 7:439.

Wiener, J., Spiro, D., Russell, P. S. (1964). An electron microscopic study of the homograft reaction. Am. J. Pathol. 44:319.

Williams, P. L., Williams, M. A., Kountz, S. L., Dempster, W. J. (1964). Ultrastructural and haemodynamic studies in canine renal transplants. J. Anat. 94:545.

Winn, H. J., Stevens, L. C., Snell, G. D. (1958). Test of alternative methods for demonstrating the histocompatibility-1 isoantigen in mice. Transplant. Bull. 5:18.

Wolfe, J. R. (1875). A new method of performing plastic operations. Br. Med. J. 2:360.

Wolff, K., Schellander, F. G. (1965). Enzyme-histochemical studies on the healing-process of split skin grafts. I. Aminopeptidase, diphosphopyridine-nucleotide-diaphorase and succinic dehydrogenase in autografts. J. Invest. Dermatol. 45:38.

Wolff, K., Schellander, F. G. (1966a). Enzyme-histochemical studies on the healing process of split skin grafts. II. 5-Nucleotidase, adenosinetriphosphatase acid and alkaline phosphatase in autografts. J. Invest. Dermatol. 46:205.

Wolff, K., Schellander, F. G. (1966b). Enzyme-histochemical studies on the healing process of split skin grafts. III. Oxidative and hydrolytic enzymes in homografts. J. Invest. Dermatol. 46:213.

Woodruff, M. F. A. (1960). The Transplantation of Tissues and Organs. Thomas, Springfield, Ill.

Woodruff, M. F. A., Simpson, L. O. (1955). Experimental skin grafting in rats. With special references to split skin grafts. Plast. Reconstr. Surg. 15:451.

Wustrack, K. O., Gruber, R. P., Lucas, Z. J. (1975). Immunological enhancement of skin allografts in the rat. Transplantation 19:156.

Yukna, R. A., Tow, H. D., Carroll, P. B., Vernino, A. R., Bright, R. W. (1977). Evaluation of the use of freeze-dried skin allografts in the treatment of human mucogingival problems. J. Periodontol. 48:187.

Yukna, R. A., Turner, D. W., Robinson, L. J. (1977). Variable antigenicity of lyophilized allogeneic and lyophilized xenogeneic skin in guinea pigs. J. Periodontal. Res. 12:197.

Zanella, G., Reif, A. E., Buenviaje, O. L., Asakuma, R., Deterling, R. A., Jr. (1968). On prolonged survival of massive skin allografts in mice. Transplantation 6:885.

Zarem, H. A., Dimitrievich, G. S. (1970). In vivo observations of the effects of Imuran on the microvasculature within full-thickness mouse skin allografts. Plast. Reconstr. Surg. 45:51.

Zarem, H. A., Zweifach, B. W., McGehee, J. M. (1967). Development of microcirculation in full thickness autogenous skin grafts in mice. Am. J. Physiol. 212:1081.

Zotikov, E. A., Budik, V. M., Puza, A. (1960). Some peculiarities of the survival time of skin homografts. Ann. N.Y. Acad. Sci. 87:166.

Zotikov, E. A., Urinson, R. M. (1962). Antigen-overloading of the recipient in the transplantation of large skin grafts. In: Mechanisms of Immunological Tolerance. Proceedings of Symposium, Liblice, Czechoslovakia. pp. 273–275.

Index